Advances in Cardiology

Vol. 31

Series Editor
J. J. Kellermann, Tel Hashomer

S. Karger · Basel · München · Paris · London · New York · Sydney

2nd World Congress on Cardiac Rehabilitation,
Jerusalem, November 30–December 3, 1981

Comprehensive Cardiac Rehabilitation

Volume Editor
J. J. Kellermann, Tel Hashomer

35 figures and 44 tables, 1982

S. Karger · Basel · München · Paris · London · New York · Sydney

Advances in Cardiology

National Library of Medicine, Cataloging in Publication
World Congress on Cardiac Rehabilitation (2nd: 1981: Jerusalem)
Comprehensive cardiac rehabilitation/
2nd World Congress on Cardiac Rehabilitation, November 30–December 3, 1981;
volume editor, J. J. Kellermann. – Basel; New York: Karger, 1982.
(Advances in cardiology; v. 31)
Organized by the Scientific Council on Cardiac Rehabilitation of the International Society and Federation of Cardiology.
1. Coronary Disease – rehabilitation – congresses 2. Myocardial Infarction – rehabilitation – congresses
I. Kellermann, Jan J. II. International Society and Federation of Cardiology. Scientific Coucil on Cardiac Rahabilitation III. Title IV. Series
W1 AD53C v. 31 [WG 300 W94 1981c]
ISBN 3–8055–3539–2

Drug Dosage

The author and publisher have exerted every effort to ensure that drug selection and dosage set forth in this text are in accord with current recommendations and practice at the time of publication. However, in view of ongoing research, changes in government regulations, and the constant flow of information relating to drug therapy and drug reactions, the reader is urged to check the package insert for each drug for any change in indications and dosage and for added warnings and precautions. This is particularly important when the recommended agent is a new and/or infrequently employed drug.

Printed in Switzerland by Merkur AG, Langenthal
ISBN 3–8055–3539–2

Contents

Preface IX

The Prognostic Significance of Exercice Stress Testing

Amsterdam, E. A.; Dressendorfer, R. H. (Davis, Calif.): Clinical Implications of Sensitivity, Specificity and Predictive Accuracy of Exercise Testing to Detect Coronary Artery Disease 1

Bruce, R. A.; Hossack, K. F.; DeRouen, T. A. (Seattle, Wash.): Prognostic Value of Exercise Testing 7

Shephard, R. J. (Toronto): Can Exercise Stress Tests Indicate Prognosis? 12

Amsterdam, E. A.; Dressendorfer, R. H. (Davis, Calif.): Value and Limitations of Exercise Testing for Detection of Coronary Artery Disease in Symptomatic and Asymptomatic Populations 19

Borer, J. S.; Phillips, P.; Moses, J. W.; Goldberg, H. L.; Fisher, J. (New York, N. Y.): Determination of Prognosis in Patients with Coronary Artery Disease by Non-invasive Radionuclide-Based Methods Applied during Exercise 23

Niederberger, M.; Gaul, G.; Schlick, W.; Wolner, E. (Wien): Prognostic Value of Exercise Testing in Respect to Effects of Aortocoronary Bypass Surgery on Functional Aerobic Capacity 28

Spodick, D. H. (Worcester, Mass.): Systolic Time Intervals: Prognostic Value and Exercise Responses 35

De Backer, G. (Gent): Prognostic Significance of Exercise-Induced Ventricular Arrhythmias in Postmyocardial Infarction Patients 38

Secondary Preventive Approach

A. Surgery

Spodick, D. H. (Worcester, Mass.): Indications for Coronary Bypass Surgery, 1982. Controlled Trials Scientifically and Ethically Optimum 45

Varnauskas, E. (Göteborg): Coronary Bypass Surgery in Prevention of Premature Mortality . . . 51
Borman, J. B.; Shimon, D. V.; Appelbaum, A.; Gotsman, M. S. (Jerusalem): Coronary Surgery as Secondary Prevention. Objectives and Achievements of Surgical Myocardial Revascularization . . . 60
Gohlke, H.; Roskamm, H.; Samek, L.; Schnellbacher, K.; Schmuziger, M. (Bad Krozingen): Long-Term Effect of Aortocoronary Bypass Surgery on Exercise Tolerance and Vocational Rehabilitation . . . 73
Wenger, N. K. (Atlanta, Ga.): Coronary Bypass Surgery as a Rehabilitative Procedure 80

B. Drugs

Julian, D. G. (Newcastle upon Tyne): Secondary Prevention after Myocardial Infarction 86
Sleight, P. (Oxford): Beta-Blockade in Acute Myocardial Infarction . . . 90
Thomas, M. (Midhurst, West Sussex): Prevention of Ischaemic Heart Disease in the Hypertensive Patient . . . 95
Van Aken, W. G. (Amsterdam): Anticoagulants and Platelet-Active Agents in the Secondary Prevention of Coronary Artery Disease . . . 98

C. Rehabilitation Programs

Denolin, H. (Bruxelles): Present and Future of Cardiac Rehabilitation . . . 102
Lamm, G.; Denolin, H.; Dorossiev, D.; Pisa, Z. (Copenhagen): Rehabilitation and Secondary Prevention of Patients after Acute Myocardial Infarction. WHO Collaborative Study . . . 107
Rost, R. (Köln): General Aspects of the Secondary Prevention of Myocardial Infarction 112
Kallio, V. (Turku): Rehabilitation Programmes as Secondary Prevention: A Community Approach . . . 120
Pollock, M. L.; Foster, C.; Rod, J. L.; Wible, G. (Milwaukee, Wisc.): Comparison of Methods for Determining Exercise Training Intensity for Cardiac Patients and Healthy Adults . . . 129
Kellermann, J. J. (Tel Hashomer): Cardiac Rehabilitation as a Secondary Preventive Measure – Endpoints. The Logic of Desirability and Availability . . . 134

Early Rehabilitation

Wenger, N. K. (Atlanta, Ga.): Early Ambulation: The Physiologic Basis Revisited . . . 138
Velasco, J. A.; Tormo, V.; Ridocci, F.; Grima, A. (Valencia): Complications during Early Ambulation and Patient Selection . . . 142
Kohn, R. M. (Buffalo, N. Y.): Early Ambulation after Myocardial Infarction. The Surgical Model . . . 147

Messin, R.; Demaret, B. (Bruxelles): Accelerated versus Classical Early Mobilization after Myocardial Infarction 152

Comprehensive Rehabilitation

DeBusk, R. F. (Stanford, Calif.): Physical Conditioning Following Myocardial Infarction 156
Kornitzer, M. (Bruxelles): Primary Coronary Risk Factors and Secondary Prevention of Coronary Heart Disease 162
Oberman, A.; Cleary, P.; Larosa, J. C.; Hellerstein, H. K.; Naughton, J. (Birmingham, Ala.): Changes in Risk Factors among Participants in a Long-Term Exercise Rehabilitation Program 168
Angster, H.; Glonner, R.; Halhuber, M. (Munich): Risk Factor Modification in the Framework of Rehabilitation. Results of a Long-Term Rehabilitation Program in Bavaria 176

Exercise as a Therapeutic Modality

Froelicher, V. (San Diego, Calif.): Exercise and Health 180
Bruce, R. A.; Hossack, K. F. (Seattle, Wash.): Rationale of Physical Training in Patients with Angina pectoris 186
Shephard, R. J. (Toronto): Exercise Therapy in Patients with Angina pectoris 191
Wenger, N. K. (Atlanta, Ga.): Is Strenuous Physical Activity Appropriate for Patients with Coronary Heart Disease? 199
Zohmann, L. R. (Bronx, N. Y.): Practical Aspects of Vigorous Exercise Programming for Coronary Patients 205

Psychological Aspects of Cardiac Rehabilitation

Hackett, T. P.; Cassem, N. H. (Boston, Mass.): Coping with Cardiac Disease 212
Acker, J. E., Jr.; MacMorran, P. R.; Friedlob, J. W.; Wade, C. C. (Knoxville, Tenn.): Assessing Psychological Problems from a Cardiologist's Point of View 218
Degré-Coustry, C.; Grévisse, M. (Bruxelles): Intensive Care Unit Members in Front of the Patients Reaction Related to an Acute Myocardial Infarction 223
Schlesinger, Z.; Segev, U. (Tel Aviv): Rehabilitation of Patients after Acute Myocardial Infarction. An Interdisciplinary Family-Oriented Program 226
Philip, A. E. (Edinburgh): Measuring the Outcome of Rehabilitation 232
Cay, E. L. (Edinburgh): Psychological Aspects of Cardiac Rehabilitation. Unsolved Problems. 237

Subject Index 242

Preface

For many years the subject of cardiac rehabilitation has been identified with physiotherapy, physical training and psychotherapy. Clinical cardiologists have viewed the rehabilitation of the cardiac patient with scepticism and doubt. However, in recent years the interest in cardiac rehabilitation is growing and very significant achievements have been made, especially since international and national institutions began to support research and cooperative studies. The Scientific Council on Cardiac Rehabilitation of the International Society and Federation of Cardiology was and is one of the most active bodies and achieved to gain worldwide recognition as one of the most productive Councils in the Society. The World Congress which took place in Hamburg in 1977 was an excellent demonstration of the efficiency of this Council, chaired for many years by Prof. *Henry Denolin* and now chaired by Prof. *Kurt Koenig.*

In organizing the Second World Congress in Jerusalem, the Scientific Committee has tried to enlarge the scope of topics to be discussed. Thus, the comprehensiveness of rehabilitative procedures was especially reflected in the scientific program. Comprehensive rehabilitation, which includes risk factor modification, exercise training and psychological and vocational counselling, must also make use of other therapeutical modalities of the cardiac patient, such as drug therapy and surgery. A close follow-up, being one of the more important clues of management of a chronic disease, enables by means of various noninvasive techniques, to reassess the clinical and functional condition of the patient repeatedly. Echocardiography, nuclear techniques and exercise testing have proved to represent very important diagnostic tools in the early detection of changes in the dynamics of the disease and thus enable the implementation of conservative or invasive therapeutic modalities. A supervised intervention program may eventually affect the prognosis and quality of survival. These programs should be considered an integrative part of coronary care.

There are still a number of unanswered questions, focused especially on the secondary preventive aspects concerning cardiac rehabilitation. Till now, a great amount of money has been invested in the organization of randomized trials, but the outcome of these studies did not disclose final conclusions as to whether or not rehabilitative procedures and especially exercise therapy, have a direct effect on morbidity and mortality. In the years ahead it will be necessary to rephrase 'slogans' change the objectives of our studies and avoid rhetoric questions and working hypotheses which cannot be proven. We should never forget that we are dealing with a multifactorial disease which must be treated by a multifactorial approach.

These, in short, were the objectives of the 2nd World Congress on Cardiac Rehabilitation, where more than 500 scientists from 31 countries participated. 48 papers were invited and presented by internationally recognized experts in their respective fields. This volume contains most of these papers.

Finally, I would like to thank all the co-sponsors especially my friends from the Scientific Council for Cardiac Rehabilitation of the ISFC, *K. Koenig* (president), *H. Denolin* (past-president) and *N. K. Wenger* (president-elect and liaison to A.H.A.). Further, the Cardiovascular Division of WHO, the American Heart Association and the Israeli Heart Society. Their assistance is most appreciated.

I should like to express my gratitude to all the speakers and last but not least to the Medical Departments of Bayer AG, Leverkusen, Imperial Chemical Industries Ltd., Cheshire, and Ciba-Geigy Ltd, Basel for their generous support.

It is my hope that the windows opened at this congress will contribute to a better understanding and enlarge the scope of cardiac rehabilitation.

Jan J. Kellermann, President,
2nd World Congress on Cardiac Rehabilitation

Adv. Cardiol., vol. 31, pp. 1–6 (Karger, Basel 1982)

Clinical Implications of Sensitivity, Specificity and Predictive Accuracy of Exercise Testing to Detect Coronary Artery Disease[1]

Ezra A. Amsterdam and Rudolph H. Dressendorfer

Division of Cardiovascular Medicine, Department of Internal Medicine, University of California School of Medicine, Davis, Calif., USA

Noninvasive screening methods have assumed increasing importance as aids in the detection of coronary artery disease. These methods can extend the clinical history through the objective data they yield and thereby facilitate early and appropriate management of the coronary patient. Although the field of noninvasive cardiology has developed at a remarkable rate during the past decade, providing new and valuable diagnostic modalities of expanded capability, the exercise test remains the most practical and widely utilized laboratory approach to identification of individuals with coronary artery disease.

Exercise ECG of Coronary Disease

Exercise testing affords diagnostic information as well as a quantitative measure of an individual's response to a controlled stress, including physical work capacity and effect on symptoms, heart rhythm and blood pressure, all of which are of potential clinical significance. However, the criteria utilized for a presumptive diagnosis of coronary artery disease by exercise testing are generally restricted to the electrocardiogram and consist of the characteristic exercise-induced alteration of the S-T segment: horizontal depression (or elevation) of 1 mm or more for 80 ms or more in an S-T segment that is normal at rest [1]. Exercise-induced alteration of the

[1] Supported by Program Project Grant HL 14780 from the National Heart, Lung and Blood Institute of the National Institutes of Health, Bethesda, Md., and California Chapters of the American Heart Association, Dallas, Tex.

electrocardiographic R wave, suggested by some as an indicator of coronary disease [2], will not be considered here. Other potential electrocardiographic indicators of exercise-induced ischemia such as alterations of the T and U waves are also under investigation. Associated electrocardiographic or clinical findings provoked by exertion (e.g. arrhythmias) may support an impression of coronary artery disease but are non-specific rather than diagnostic and may be associated with non-coronary cardiac disease. In this regard, exercise-induced S-T segment depression is also not indicative of a single diagnostic entity, i.e. coronary artery disease, but rather should be viewed as presumptive evidence of stress-related myocardial ischemia, which may be associated with a number of cardiac abnormalities, in addition to coronary disease, that can produce a disparity between myocardial oxygen supply and demand (e.g. aortic valve disease). This finding can also occur, for unknown reasons, in the absence of any detectable abnormality of the heart and coronary circulation. It is important to emphasize that the results of exercise testing must always be evaluated as only one set of data in the total context of a patient's assessment.

Definitions of Diagnostic Test Results

For the sole purpose of diagnosing coronary artery disease, the utility of exercise electrocardiography can be expressed by a number of terms reflecting different aspects of the test results, as defined in table I. It is noted that each of the terms in table I conveys different information. *Sensitivity* and *specificity* indicate the proportion of subjects with and without a disease, respectively, that can be accurately identified by a test. Of perhaps more immediate relevance to the clinician, *predictive accuracy* shows the proportion of results that is correct among the positive and negative test outcomes.

Relation of Exercise ECG to Coronary Angiography

Selective coronary angiography has been a conventional standard of reference on which are based the sensitivity, specificity and predictive accuracy of exercise electrocardiography for the detection of coronary artery disease. Alternatively, long-term epidemiologic follow-up studies, with correlation between test results and substantiation of coronary disease

Table I. Definition of terms used to evaluate the accuracy of diagnostic tests

Sensitivity (%)	= Percent of all subjects with a disease in whom the test for that disease is positive (true-positive; TP) (False-negative [FN] is a negative result of the test in a subject with the disease) $= \frac{TP}{TP+FN} \times 100$ or $\frac{TP}{\text{All subjects with the disease}} \times 100$
Specificity (%)	= Percent of all subjects without the disease in whom the test is negative (true-negative, TN). (False-positive [FP] is a positive result of the test in a subject without the disease) $= \frac{TN}{TN+FP} \times 100$ or $\frac{TN}{\text{All subjects without the disease}} \times 100$
Predictive accuracy of a positive test (%)	= Percent of all subjects with a positive test (TP+FP) who have the disease (TP) $= \frac{TP}{TP+FP} \times 100$ or $\frac{TP}{\text{All subjects with a positive test}} \times 100$
Predictive accuracy of a negative test (%)	= Percent of all subjects with a negative test for a disease (TN+FN) who do not have the disease (TN) $= \frac{TN}{TN+FN} \times 100$ or $\frac{TN}{\text{All subjects with a negative test}} \times 100$

by development of coronary events, have also been applied to assess the utility of diagnostic exercise electrocardiography [3]. The latter approach has been chiefly utilized in the asymptomatic population in which invasive evaluation is not feasible.

The limitations of and problems posed by comparison of disparate techniques such as exercise electrocardiography and coronary angiography for detection of coronary artery disease are appreciable. Angiography is an anatomic method based on measurement of static abnormalities and exercise electrocardiography attempts to identify a dynamic, physiologic deficit. Thus, uniformity should not be anticipated in a comparison of the findings of these two methods. However, such problems notwithstanding, coronary angiography has provided a reasonable means of evaluating the accuracy of methods employed to detect clinically important coronary artery disease. It is on the basis of angiographically determined coronary artery disease that clinical course and, thus, patient management are determined [4]. Further, in vitro anatomic data demonstrate satisfactory correlation with angiographic assessment of coronary pathoanatomy [5].

Diagnostic Accuracy of Exercise Electrocardiography

Many studies have been published indicating the sensitivity, specificity and predictive accuracy of exercise electrocardiography in the diagnosis of coronary artery disease [1]. When coronary artery disease is defined as the presence of 70% or greater narrowing of coronary luminal diameter in one or more major coronary arteries and the criterion of 1.0mm or greater S-T segment depression for 80ms or more is utilized to define a positive test, the sensitivity of exercise electrocardiography for detection of the disease is approximately 70% and its specificity is approximately 90%. Obviously, less stringent criteria for a positive test result (e.g. 0.5mm S-T segment depression) would yield a higher sensitivity (more true positives) but lower specificity (more false positives). Conversely, stricter criteria for a positive result (e.g. 2.0mm S-T segment depression) would decrease sensitivity (fewer true positives) but would raise specificity (fewer false positives). An extremely important factor determining sensitivity is extent of coronary artery disease. Sensitivities for one, two and three vessel coronary artery disease are approximately 45%, 65% and 85%, respectively [1]. It should be emphasized that utilization of exercise electrocardiography to detect coronary artery disease is predicated on performance of a meaningful exercise test, which can be generally defined as achievement of at least 85% of a patient's age-predicted maximum effort, unless criteria for discontinuation of the test occur at an earlier stage of the study.

Effect of Disease Prevalence on Test Results – Bayes' Theorem

A major advance in understanding the results of exercise electrocardiography has been, as stated in *Bayes'* [6] theorem, the concept that test outcome is not only a function of the sensitivity and specificity of the method, but also of the prevalence of the disease in the population under investigation. This concept is of considerable importance, since exercise electrocardiography is being increasingly applied as a screening procedure for coronary disease in asymptomatic groups, in which disease prevalence is

Table II. Relation of the test results to prevalence of disease and to sensitivity (70%) and specificity (90%) of test (1,000 subjects)

		Positive exercise ECG	Negative exercise ECG
Consider disease prevalence 90%			
Normal (10%)	100	90 (10% false-positive)	10 (90% true-negative)
CAD (90%)	900	630 (70% true-positive)	270 (30% false-negative)
Total	1,000	720	280
Consider disease prevalence 5%			
Normal (95%)	950	95 (10% false-positive)	855 (90% true-negative)
CAD (5%)	50	35 (70% true-positive)	15 (30% false-negative)
Total	1,000	130	870

CAD = Coronary artery disease.

usually very low. The predictive accuracy of the test result obtained by the clinician is highly dependent on the pretest probability of the presence of disease, as is illustrated by the following examples.

Table II depicts the predictive accuracy of a positive test result in a population of patients with clinical evidence of coronary disease, suggested, for example, by a history of typical angina pectoris. It is known that the presence of the latter confers a pretest probability of the presence of coronary disease of approximately 90% [7]. Thus, with a test of 70% sensitivity and 90% specificity, 87% of the positive responses will be true ones and there will be relatively few false-positive results. On the other hand, the predictive accuracy of a positive test in a subject with a low pretest probability of disease is quite different, as indicated in table II, even though the sensitivity and specificity of the method are unchanged. Thus in this example, only about one of four positive results is true-positive and a majority is false-positive. Great care must therefore be taken in interpreting and acting upon positive test results in asymptomatic populations. Aid in interpretation can be obtained by considering the result as one factor in total patient evaluation and assessing the finding in terms of the total coronary risk profile. Further, factors of general application in enhancing the predictive accuracy of positive exercise electrocardiographic results include marked ($\geq$ 2.0 mm) S-T segment alteration, ischemic S-T segment change at low heart rate ($\leq$ 80% of predicted maximum) or at an early stage of exercise ($\leq$ 3 min), ischemic changes in multiple electrocardiographic leads and prolonged duration ($\geq$ 5 min) of ischemic S-T segment depression during postexercise recovery [8].

References

1 Silverman, M. E.; Silverman, B. D.: The diagnostic capabilities and limitations of the electrocardiogram, pp. 13–45; in Hurst, Update II: the heart. Bypass surgery for obstructive coronary disease (McGraw-Hill, New York 1980).

2 Bonoris, P. E.; Greenberg, P. S.; Christison, G. W.; Castellanet, M. J.; Ellestad, M. H.: Evaluation of R wave amplitude changes versus S-T segment depression in stress testing. Circulation *57:* 904–910 (1978).

3 Amsterdam, E. A.; Mason, D. T.: Prognostic importance of exercise tests, pp. 183–193; in James, Amsterdam, Coronary heart disease, exercise testing and cardiac rehabilitation (Symposia Specialists Medical Books, Miami 1977).

4 Bruschke, A. V. G.; Proudfit, W. L.; Sones, F. M.: Progress study of 590 consecutive nonsurgical cases of coronary disease followed 5–9 years. 1. Arteriographic correlations. Circulation *47:* 1147–1153 (1973).

5 Kemp, H. G.; Evans, H.; Elliott, W. C.; Gorlin, R.: Diagnostic accuracy of selective coronary cinearteriography. Circulation *36:* 526–533 (1967).

6 Bayes, T.: An essay toward solving a problem in the doctrine of chance. Phil. Trans. R. Soc. *53:* 370 (1963).

7 Laslett, L. J.; Amsterdam, E. A.; Mason, D. T.: Evaluating the positive exercise stress test in the asymptomatic individual. Chest (in press).

8 Amsterdam, E. A.; Dressendorfer, R. H.; Mason, D. T.: Toward improved interpretation of the exercise test. Cardiology *66:* 236–240 (1980).

Prof. E. A. Amsterdam, MD, Division of Cardiovascular Medicine, School of Medicine, University of California, Davis, CA 95616 (USA)

Adv. Cardiol., vol. 31, pp. 7–11 (Karger, Basel 1982)

Prognostic Value of Exercise Testing[1]

R. A. Bruce, K. F. Hossack, T. A. DeRouen

Divisions of Cardiology and Biostatistics, University of Washington, Seattle, Wash., USA

Introduction

Symptom-limited multistage treadmill testing of exercise responses enhances assessment of prognosis [1–4] in ambulatory healthy persons or patients with chronic cardiovascular diseases seen in office or clinical practice. The functional limits of the cardiovascular system are defined in relation to symptoms, physical and ECG signs, and three important, noninvasive measurements, namely duration of exercise (by *Bruce*'s protocol), heart rate and systolic pressure. These variables may be interpreted in relation to normal standards adjusted for sex, age, and habitual activity status. 10 years' experience with this method in community practice involving several scores of physicians has demonstrated its feasibility and acceptance.

Materials and Methods

Data on 6,650 persons with maximal exercise test results and an average follow-up for 7 years were reviewed in relation to coronary heart disease (CHD) morbidity and mortality events reported by periodic mail questionnaire and other records. Overall crude mortality was 8.1%, and persons withdrawn or lost to follow-up made up 8.4%. Age-standardized event rates for each clinical group were computed from the number of first events per 1,000 person-years of observation from time of initial testing. Differences in rates indicate component risks attributable to conventional risk factors, salient clinical evidence of heart disease, various exercise indicators and pathophysiological syndromes of exertional myocardial ischemia and left-ventricular dysfunction.

[1] Supported by grants and contracts from the National Heart, Lung and Blood Institute, Bethesda, Md.

Table I. Incidence

	Healthy	Hypertensive	Atypical chest pain
Primary events (1,000 men/year; age standardized)			
CHD morbidity	4.5 (4.4)	9.6 (8.8)	9.5 (10.8)
CHD mortality	0.9 (0.0)	4.1 (1.0)	0.4 (0.0)
Both morbidity and mortality	5.4 (4.4)	13.7 (9.8)	9.9 (10.8)
Total events in relation to risk factors, exercise responses			
No risk factor, no exercise predictor	3.2 (2.5)	8.7 (0.0)	3.2 (10.7)
Only risk factor	5.2 (6.1)	13.1 (3.1)	7.5 (6.3)
Only exercise predictor	3.9 (0.0)	13.7 (4.6)	14.9 (10.7)
Risk factor and exercise predictor	*12.6* (7.9)	*34.6* (13.1)	*22.6* (7.7)

Figures in parentheses are values obtained for women.

Results

Symptom-Limited Maximal Exercise Testing

Ages ranged from 19 to 84 (48.1±8.9) years in 5,709 men, and from 23 to 78 (50.7±8.9) years in women. The highest age-specific incidence of primary CHD events in healthy men was 9/1,000 person-years in men of 55–64 years of age. For men with CHD syndromes (i.e., angina pectoris, prior myocardial infarction, or sudden cardiac arrest with resuscitation by ventricular defibrillation, whether or not in association with hypertension), the age-specific incidence of secondary CHD events approximated 78/1,000 person-years from ages 30 to 59 years. The major question is whether risk factors, clinical findings and exercise test responses enhance risk assessment over these event rates established retrospectively.

Annual event rates for 2,556 healthy men [2] and women, 873 patients with hypertension [4] and 697 patients with atypical chest pain syndromes (specifically not angina pectoris) are presented in table I.

Hypertension (however defined by each physician, and whether or not already treated) and atypical chest pain syndromes increase the risks of CHD events. Higher event rates are observed in men than in women, except for women with atypical chest pain syndromes. The highest risk

Table II. Incidence of 'hard' events in CHD patients (see text)

	Incidence
Secondary events (1,000 men/year; age standardized)	
Morbidity (myocardial infarction)	15.0 (21.4)
Mortality (sudden cardiac death, nonsudden cardiac death)	24.8 (24.6)
Both morbidity and mortality	39.8 (46.0)
Total events in relation to exercise responses	
Neither exertional myocardial ischemia nor left-ventricular dysfunction	30.0 (15.3)
Only exertional myocardial ischemia	46.2 (11.3)
Only left-ventricular dysfunction	110.0 (81.0)
Both exertional myocardial ischemia and left-ventricular dysfunction	97.3 (46.5)

Figures in parentheses are values obtained for women.

occurs with the interaction of one or more conventional risk factors (i.e., family history of myocardial infarction or sudden cardiac death, smoking of cigarettes, hypertension of ≥140 mm Hg systolic pressure and/or hypercholesterolemia of 250 mg/dl or higher) and two or more exercise predictors [2]. In healthy men, four such predictors have been identified, namely, chest pain with maximal exercise testing, exercise duration of less than 6 min, peak heart rate less than 90% of age-predicted normal value, and/or one or more millimeters of ischemic ST depression [2]. In hypertensive men, the other risk factors, and especially risk factor tally, are significant, but ischemic ST depression is not [4]. Peak heart rate under 80% of predicted and functional aerobic impairment of 25% or more are predictors [4].

More recent data for secondary 'hard' CHD events in CHD patients [3] are shown in table II. These are defined as myocardial infarction, sudden cardiac arrest/resuscitation or cardiac death to eliminate hospitalizations for study of angina or treatment by coronary bypass surgery as a possible consequence of responses to exercise testing.

Secondary CHD event rates are higher than primary CHD events. Morbidity rate in 1,956 men is less than that in a sample of 369 women; yet mortality rates for the two sexes are identical. Total 'hard' events range from 30/1,000 men with neither exertional pathophysiological syndrome to 110/1,000 men in those with only left-ventricular dysfunction. The later is defined by one or more noninvasive variables, namely cardiomegaly, exercise duration less than 3 min, or peak systolic pressure with exercise less than 130 mm Hg. Patients also with exertional myocardial ischemia (i.e.

chest pain with maximal exercise and/or ischemic ST depression) exhibit lower risk rates. Lower event rates are observed with these exercise predictors in women than in men.

Use of these pathophysiological syndromes as possible guidelines was evaluated in relation to 4-year survival of 2,001 CHD men who were treated either medically or surgically [1]. In retrospect, patients with only exertional myocardial ischemia (the usually accepted clinical criterion for surgery) showed an insignificant difference in 4-year survival (92 vs. 91%). 34% of the patients with left-ventricular dysfunction, with or without myocardial ischemia, who were operated on had a 94% survival in contrast to 67% survival for the medically treated patients who had at least one coronary artery graftable ($p < 0.01$). This suggests the value of noninvasive exercise testing to screen patients for invasive diagnostic studies, and, if indicated, bypass surgical treatment.

Discussion and Conclusions

Multistage treadmill testing of maximal exercise responses extend clinical evaluation of middle-aged persons. Symptom-limited testing, in the absence of acute illness or contraindications, safely defines functional limits of the cardiovascular system and identifies major mechanisms of cardiac impairment which may be quantitatively assessed in relation to appropriate normal standards. Whereas several exercise predictors enhance prognosis for either primary or secondary CHD events, the major emphasis many physicians place on ST responses is not adequately justified. Although an important marker of imbalance between oxygen supply and left-ventricular demand, it is nonspecific, and in the absence of conventional risk factors or salient clinical manifestations of heart disease, it is frequently misleading with respect to prognosis as well as diagnosis.

References

1 Bruce, R. A.; DeRouen, T. A.; Hammermeister, K.: Noninvasive screening criteria for enhanced 4-year survival after aortocoronary bypass surgery. Circulation *60:* 638–646 (1979).

2 Bruce, R. A.; DeRouen, T. A.; Hossack, K. F.: Value of maximal exercise tests in risk assessment of primary coronary heart disease events in healthy men. Five years experience on the Seattle Heart Watch. Am. J. Cardiol. *46:* 371–378 (1980).

3 Bruce, R. A.; DeRouen, T. A.; Peterson, D. R.; Irving, J. B.; Chinn, N.; Blake, B.; Hofer, V.: Non-invasive predictors of sudden cardiac death in man with coronary heart disease. Predictive value of maximal exercise stress testing. Am. J. Cardiol. *39:* 833–840 (1977).

4 Hossack, K. F.; Bruce, R. A.; DeRouen, T. A.: Evaluation of hypertensive males for primary coronary heart disease events using conventional risk factors and maximal exercise testing. Clin. Cardiol. *3:* 229–235 (1980).

R. A. Bruce, MD, University Hospital, Division of Cardiology, RG-20,
University of Washington, Seattle, WA 98195 (USA)

Adv. Cardiol., vol. 31, pp. 12–18 (Karger, Basel 1982)

Can Exercise Stress Tests Indicate Prognosis?

Roy J. Shephard

School of Physical and Health Education, Department of Preventive Medicine and Biostatistics and Institute of Medical Sciences and Toronto Rehabilitation Centre, Toronto, Ont., Canada

The Problem of Misclassification

> 'The augmented two-step test, when negative, completely excludes the presence of coronary artery disease'
>
> *Master* [21]

Unfortunately, few of the current generation of cardiologists can accept *Master's* statement. A proportion of subjects with normal prognosis develop substantial ST segmental depression during a stress test, and a proportion of patients with a poor prognosis show an apparently normal response.

Reference Standard. The assessment of the prognostic value of a stress test implies some absolute reference standard against which judgement can be made. Unfortunately, there is no simple and unequivocal indicator of cardiac prognosis.

Many reports compare stress results to angiography, rather than to the clinical prognosis as seen by prospective study. Intraobserver variation in the interpretation of angiograms is substantial [11, 29]. In a proportion of false-positive diagnoses, the angiogram shows a minor (30–50%) obstruction, but this has been dismissed as clinically insignificant [13]. Moreover, because of the risks of angiography, it is rarely possible to check the validity of a negative exercise ECG. Angiograms generally overstate the number of positive tests relative to a moderate period of clinical observation. Time converts a proportion of false-positive to true-positive results, but unfortunately there is also a larger increase in the number of false-negative stress test reports.

Test Sensitivity. The sensitivity measures the completeness with which a test detects abnormal individuals. It can be increased by reducing the severity of the abnormal criterion, but the penalty is then an increase in the proportion of false-positive tests.

Test Specificity. The specificity indicates the precision with which normality is recognized. It can be improved by setting a more stringent criterion of abnormality, but the penalty is then a loss of sensitivity [20].

Setting the Criterion. The choice of test sensitivity and specificity should be influenced by such factors as the cost of a false-positive diagnosis, the seriousness of a false-negative diagnosis, the intended frequency of screening and the prevalence of the disease within the community. A false-positive stress test may expose a patient to the unnecessary expense and danger of an angiogram, and create iatrogenic disability. A false-negative diagnosis is perhaps the lesser of two evils, although it may encourage excessively strenuous physical activity and weaken the impact of advice concerning an adverse life-style.

The prevalence of abnormal exercise ECGs in the general population rises from near zero at age 30 to about 20% at age 65 years. Thus, a fairly high test sensitivity is needed in order to yield a useful proportion of positive results when screening ostensibly healthy individuals. However, a lesser sensitivity is acceptable if the test is to be performed annually. Abnormalities missed at the first examination will then be detected in subsequent years.

Design of Screening Programmes

Optimum Test Protocol. The sensitivity and specificity of the stress ECG are improved by: (a) carrying out near-maximum rather than low intensity exercise; (b) use of multiple rather than single ECG leads, and (c) recording both during and following exercise.

Additional prognostic information can be derived from the intensity of exercise provoking ST depression [13], the contour of the ST depression into the recovery period, and concordance between exercise and recovery records [6]. If a 12-lead ECG is recorded during exercise to 85% of maximum effort and during recovery, the sensitivity relative to angiography is about 80%, while the specificity is around 90% [1].

Screening a Normal Population. If such a test is applied to 1,000 people from a population with a 5% prevalence of ischemic heart disease, more than 10% of patients are wrongly classified. More than 70% of warnings of an adverse prognosis are incorrect (95 false-positive tests) and 10 patients are also given false-negative reports.

Surprisingly, these statistics are quite compatible with reports that a positive stress test indicates a 2 to 15-fold worsening of prognosis [1, 9, 13]. Indeed, in the example cited, the average outlook is 25 times worse for those individuals with a positive stress test. Nevertheless, a much greater test specificity is needed. Even if we could develop a screening test with a specificity of 98%, at least a third of ostensibly healthy middle-aged adults would be wrongly warned of impending cardiac disease.

Selective Screening. A more practical alternative is to restrict the application of screening to patients with a high risk of ischemic heart disease. The likelihood of cardiac disease could be increased 8.5-fold if the examination were restricted to patients with a combination of a low energy output, heavy cigarette smoking, and a high resting systolic blood pressure [22]. In such a sample, the total percentage of patients misclassified by a stress test would increase slightly (to 14.3%), but less than 15% of the supposed adverse prognoses would be erroneous. Because of this marked influence of disease prevalence, ECG screening is much more effective in elderly than in younger populations [16]. It is particularly helpful in identifying critical lesions, picking out as many as 92% of patients with left main stem disease [10].

Bayes Theorem. Bayes theorem allows a more formal calculation of the prognostic value of the exercise ECG. In populations with a low prevalence of ischemic heart disease, the tossing of a coin is superior to exercise testing [15, 17]. As disease prevalence increases, the information content of a positive test improves, while that of a negative test deteriorates. Given a 20% prevalence of disease, the baseline expectation of abnormality is 20%, the information yield of a positive response is 46.7%, and that of a negative response is 14.7%.

One flaw in the direct application of Bayes theorem is that the sensitivity and specificity of the test are assumed to be independent of the severity of the disease; in practice, sensitivity is increased substantially if there is 2- or 3-vessel disease.

Screening after Infarction. In the postcoronary patient, test sensitivity (41%) and specificity (78%) are poorer than before infarction [19]; over a 3-year period of observation, a negative test is correct in 94% of instances, but a positive test is incorrect in 88%.

Suboptimal Conditions. The statistics cited thus far refer to optimal conditions, but during mass screening the sensitivity and specificity may be even poorer. Tachycardia, hyperventilation, and lack of warm-up can all give false-positive results, while a negative result may reflect an inadequate intensity of exercise (poor motivation, clinical concerns, or extracardiac symptoms) rather than the absence of disease. False-positive results are particularly frequent in female patients [9, 25].

Causes of Erroneous Test Results

False-Positive Results. False-positive results may be traced to various drugs (digitalis, procaine amide, quinidine, antihypertensives, or antidepressants), potassium loss, cigarette smoking, carbohydrate loading, resting ST abnormalities, conduction abnormalities, left ventricular stress, cardiac hypertrophy, valvular heart disease and congestive myopathy. False-negative results can arise from use of drugs (propranolol, nitroglycerine), resting ST elevation, abnormalities of ventricular conduction, and insufficient exercise [23, 30].

Reliability of ECG Interpretation. Bailey et al. [2] found that 4% of subjects cleared by a standard exercise stress test developed an abnormal ECG when the test was repeated a few days later. *Cumming* [9] found 18% of abnormal records disappeared with repeat testing, and *Bruce* et al. [7] set the proportion of resolved abnormalities as high as 58%.

Variability of interpretation is even greater if several observers are involved [5]. Interestingly, well-trained technicians give more reliable data than cardiologists, with complete interobserver agreement in 85% of tracings; indeed, in patients with >1 mm of ST depression, they are unanimous in detecting this sign. Reliability is helped by (a) standard instructions, (b) use of a magnifying lens, and (c) period checks of performance against known ECG records.

Improving Test Accuracy

Alternative Procedures. Clinical assessment often offers a surprisingly good alternative to stress testing [9, 14, 24]. Given a typical history of angina, there is 90–95% agreement with coronary angiography. In atypical angina, agreement drops to 60%, but in nonanginal pain there is again 90–95% agreement with the criterion. Thus, in a randomly selected population, clinical examination has a sensitivity of about 90%, with a specificity of 75–80%.

The most promising of other alternative approaches are ^{201}Tl scintigraphy and radionuclide angiography, both being carried out immediately after vigorous exercise [2, 3, 18]. Some reports indicate a high sensitivity and specificity for such tests, although to date most of the available information has been collected on patients with a high probability of coronary vascular disease.

Following infarction, the one simple observation that has fair prognostic value is exercise compliance. Subjects unwilling to adhere to an exercise rehabilitation programme have a 23-fold increase in the risk of recurrent disease.

Other possibilities for the future are (a) to use the patient as his own control [8, 12, 26], comparing data with previous annual stress tests, and (b) the application of multivariate and discriminant function techniques [4, 6, 16, 27, 28].

The Role of Stress Testing

Despite strong indictments [9], there remain several potential justifications for carrying out an exercise stress test [13]. Two merit serious consideration.

(1) *Definition of a 'safe' level of exercise.* Although this approach has many advocates, it is beset by criticisms of poor test reliability, false-positive and false-negative results; further the defined safe intensity depends markedly upon incidental details of the exercise to be undertaken. Possibly, these objections can be overcome, at least in part by relating exercise prescriptions to the cardiac work-rate, as estimated from the pulse-pressure product [13].

(2) *Motivation.* The mystique of the laboratory test can have a profound effect upon the physician and the patient, providing both a prop

to a shaky diagnosis and strong motivation to a change of life-style. Whether cheaper and safer exercise protocols would provide the same psychological rewards has yet to be determined.

References

1 Ascoop, C. A.: What is an abnormal ischemic ECG response to exercise? in James, Amsterdam, Coronary heart disease, exercise testing and cardiac rehabilitation, pp. 143–154 (Symposia Specialists, Miami 1977).

2 Bailey, I. K.; Griffith, L. S. C.; Rouleau, J., et al.: Thallium 201 myocardial perfusion imaging at rest and during exercise. Circulation *55:* 79–87 (1977).

3 Berger, B. C.; Watson, D. D.; Taylor, G. J.; Craddock, G. B.; Martin, R. P.; Bellar, G. A.: Sensitivity of quantitative thallium 201 scintigraphy following nondiagnostic exercise stress. Circulation *59/60:* suppl. II, p. 172 (1979).

4 Berman, J. L.; Wynne, J.; Cohn, P. F.: Multiple-lead QRS changes with exercise testing: diagnostic value and hemodynamic implications. Circulation *61:* 53–61 (1980).

5 Blackburn, H.: The exercise electrocardiogram: technological, procedural and conceptual developments; in Blackburn, Measurement in exercise electrocardiography. The Ernst Simonson Conference (Thomas, Springfield 1969).

6 Blackburn, H.: The exercise electrocardiogram in diagnosis. Cardiology *62:* 190–205 (1977).

7 Bruce, R. A.; Pas, Y. L.; Ting, N., et al.: Seven year follow-up of cardiovascular study and maximal exercise of Chinese men. Circulation *51:* 890–901 (1975).

8 Bruce, R. A.: Exercise electrocardiography; in Hurst, The heart; 3rd ed. (McGraw-Hill, New York 1970).

9 Cumming, G. R.: Resolve that the exercise electrocardiogram is of limited diagnostic value; in Landry, Orban, Sports medicine, pp. 13–29 (Symposia Specialists, Miami 1978).

10 Dagenais, G. R.; Irshad, F.: The diagnostic value of exercise electrocardiogram: a five year experience; in Landry, Orban, Sports medicine, pp. 31–39 (Symposia Specialists, Miami 1978).

11 Detré, K. M.; Wright, E.; Murphy, M. L., et al.: Observer agreement in evaluating coronary angiograms. Circulation *52:* 979–986 (1975).

12 Doyle, J. T.; Kinch, S. H.: The prognosis of an abnormal electrocardiographic stress test. Circulation *41:* 545–553 (1970).

13 Ellestad, M. H.; Halliday, W. K.: Stress testing in the prognosis and management of ischemic heart disease. Angiology *28:* 149–159 (1977).

13 Erikssen, J.; Enge, I.; Forgang, K.; Storstein, O.: False positive diagnostic tests and coronary angiographic findings in 105 presumably healthy males. Circulation *54:* 371–376 (1981).

15 Froelicher, V. F.; Yanovitz, F. G.; Thompson, A. J.; Lancaster, M. C.: The correlation of coronary arteriography and the electrocardiographic response to maximal treadmill testing in 76 asymptomatic men. Circulation *48:* 597–604 (1973).

16 Froelicher, V. F.: Use of the exercise electrocardiogram to identify latent atherosclerotic

heart disease; in Amsterdam, Wilmore, DeMaria, Exercise in cardiovascular health and disease (Yorke Medical Books, New York 1977).

17 Goldschlager, N.; Selzer, A.; Cohn, K.: Treadmill stress tests as indicators of presence and severity of coronary artery disease. Ann. intern. Med. *85:* 277–286 (1976).

18 Johnstone, D. E.; Sands, M. J.; Berger, H. J.; Reduto, L. A.; Lachman, A. S.; Wackers, F. J. T.; Cohen L. S.; Gottschalk, A.; Zaret, B. L.; Pytlik, L.: Comparison of exercise radionucleide angiography and thallium 201 myocardial perfusion imaging in coronary artery disease. Am. J. Cardiol. *45:* 1113–1119 (1980).

19 Kavanagh, T.; Shephard, R. J.; Chisholm, A. W.; Qureshi, S.; Kennedy, J.: Prognostic indices for ischemic heart disease patients enrolled in an exercise-centred rehabilitation programme. Am. J. Cardiol. *44:* 1230–1240 (1979).

20 Martin, C. M.; McConahay, D. R.: Maximal treadmill exercise electrocardiography. Circulation *46:* 956–962 (1972).

21 Master, A. M.: Exercise testing for evaluation of cardiac performance. Am. J. Cardiol. *30:* 718–721 (1972).

22 Paffenbarger R.: Physical activity and fatal heart attack. Protection or selection? In Amsterdam, Wilmore, Exercise in cardiovascular health and disease (Yorke Medical Books, New York 1977).

23 Piessens, J.; Van Mieghem, W.; Kestelost, H.; DeGeest, H.: Diagnostic value of clinical history, exercise testing and atrial pacing in patients with chest pain. Am. J. Cardiol. *33:* 351–356 (1974).

24 Redwood, D. R.; Epstein, S. E.: Uses and limitations of stress testing in the evaluation of ischemic heart disease. Circulation *46:* 1115–1131 (1972).

25 Shephard, R. J.: Physical activity and aging (Croom Helm, London 1978).

26 Shephard, R. J.; Turner, M. E.: On the probability of correct diagnosis by pulmonary function tests. Thorax *14:* 300–304 (1959).

27 Siegel, W.: New perspectives in clinical exercise testing; in Landry, Orban, Sports medicine, pp. 3–12 (Symposia Specialists, Miami 1978).

28 Simoons, M. L.; Hugenholz, P. G.: Estimation of the probability of exercise-induced ischemia by quantitative ECG analysis. Circulation *56:* 552–559 (1979).

29 Zir, L. M.; Miller, S. W.; Dinsmore, R. E., et al.: Interobserver variability in coronary angiography. Circulation *51/52:* suppl. II, p. 27 (1975).

30 Zohman, L. R.; Kattus, A. A.: Exercise testing in the diagnosis of coronary heart disease: a perspective. Am. J. Cardiol. *40:* 243–250 (1977).

Dr. R. Shephard, 320 Huron Street, Toronto, Ont. M5S 1A1 (Canada)

Adv. Cardiol., vol. 31, pp. 19–22 (Karger, Basel 1982)

Value and Limitations of Exercise Testing for Detection of Coronary Artery Disease in Symptomatic and Asymptomatic Populations[1]

Ezra A. Amsterdam and Rudolph H. Dressendorfer

Division of Cardiovascular Medicine, Department of Internal Medicine, University of California School of Medicine, Davis, Calif., USA

Exercise testing is an important component in the evaluation of patients with symptomatic coronary artery disease (CAD) and is of potential importance in the identification of asymptomatic individuals with occult CAD. Exercise testing may provide information of importance in regard to the presence of the disease, the extent of coronary involvement and prognosis. In both symptomatic and asymptomatic populations, optimum utilization of this diagnostic method is predicated on an understanding of its value and limitations. Above all, the exercise test (ET) should always be considered as one aspect of the total patient evaluation and applied as such in clinical decision making.

Identification of CAD

The sensitivity of the diagnostic ET in the detection of CAD is approximately 70% and its specificity is approximately 90% [1]; that is, 70% of patients with CAD will have characteristic ischemic ST-segment depression of ≥1 mm for ≥80 ms induced by an adequate ET and 90% of normal individuals will have a negative response. Thus, about 30% of coronary patients will not be identified by exercise testing because of false-negative results and 10% of normal subjects will have positive tests. The sensitivity of the ET is directly related to the severity of CAD: approxi-

[1] Supported by Program Project grant HL 14780 from the National Heart, Lung and Blood Institute of the National Institutes of Health, Bethesda, Md. and California Chapters of the American Heart Association, Dallas, Tex.

Table I. Potential causes of a false-positive exercise test and a false-negative exercise test

False-positive exercise test
Pre-existent ST-segment abnormality of any cause
Drugs (digitalis, diuretics, psychoactive agents)
Electrolyte abnormality
Non-fasting state
Vasoregulatory asthenia
Occurrence of positive test only at near maximum or maximum heart rate
False-negative exercise test
Inadequate level of exertion
Effective antianginal therapy
Use of only single ECG lead

mately 45% in 1-vessel CAD, 65% in 2-vessel CAD and 85% in 3-vessel CAD [1]. Thus although there is a relatively high rate of false-negative results, exercise testing tends to selectively identify patients with more serious CAD.

It has been noted by some investigators that females tend to have a higher frequency of false-positive ETs than males but this is not invariably so [1]. Indeed our own data, based on correlative coronary angiography in a total of 161 men and women, demonstrated a false-positive ET rate of 11% in the males and 15% in the females, a statistically insignificant difference. There are multiple causes of false-positive and false-negative findings (table I) which must be considered in interpreting the ET.

The predictive accuracy of a positive ET varies greatly between symptomatic and asymptomatic populations. This disparity is related to the considerable difference in disease prevalence in these two groups and can be explained by Bayes' theorem. This issue is considered elsewhere [*Amsterdam and Dressendorfer,* this volume]. Factors that increase the predictive accuracy of positive ET results in the symptomatic population include exercise-induced ST-segment depression that occurs at a low heart rate or workload, and is marked, downsloping, present in multiple leads and prolonged post-exercise [2]. Additional supportive data include the occurrence of anginal-type chest discomfort, arrhythmias and inadequate blood pressure response during the ET. Many of these factors may also be helpful in enhancing the predictive accuracy of a positive ET in asymptomatic individuals. It is our current practice to perform rest and exercise thallium myocardial perfusion scintigraphy as part of the diagnostic evaluation when indicated in asymptomatic subjects with positive ETs. This procedure has a considerably lower rate of false-positive results than the ET [3].

Relation to Extent of CAD

Recent findings have demonstrated that the ET can provide important data regarding the extent of CAD. Marked, exercise-induced ST-segment depression is highly predictive of, in addition to the presence of CAD, severe multivessel or left main coronary involvement [2]. Thus, ≥3 mm ST-segment depression was associated with CAD in all of 37 patients, of whom 25% had left main coronary disease and 95% left anterior descending coronary disease [4]. Similarly, ST-segment depression of ≥4 mm correlated highly with the presence of left main or multivessel CAD [5].

The negative ET, while not excluding CAD, may identify patients with a low probability of severe, extensive coronary lesions and thus with a potentially good prognosis. Thus, there is less than a 10% probability of the presence of 3-vessel CAD associated with the achievement of stage III of the Bruce exercise protocol [1]. Further, of 53 patients evaluated for chest pain, all of whom had negative exercise tests, ≥85% of predicted maximal heart rate, none had left main or 3-vessel CAD [6]. In another study of more than 1,400 patients, the prevalence of 3-vessel and left main CAD in the negative ET group was 15 and 1%, respectively, compared to 73 and 27% in subjects with a positive test in the first 3 min of exercise [7].

Relation to Prognosis

The initial demonstration by *Robb and Marks* [8] that the degree of exercise-induced ST-segment depression predicted the relative risk of cardiac mortality has been confirmed and extended by recent studies [9] linking ET data to the extent of CAD, and the latter to prognosis in CAD. In patients with angiographically documented CAD, the ET has identified high and low prognostic risk, those individuals with negative ETs having a 4-year survival of 90% compared to 77% in the group with positive tests [7]. A recent innovative application of ET has been in the early period following acute myocardial infarction. In this setting, low intensity testing has identified subsequent prognostic risk, as indicated by the report of

Theroux et al. [10] in which an ischemic ET response was associated with a 1-year mortality of 27% compared with a 2.1% death rate in the negative ET group. Non-electrocardiographic findings provoked by exercise testing also may be of important prognostic value. Thus, inadequate blood pressure response (systolic <130 mm Hg) and inability to complete stage I of the Bruce exercise protocol correlated with more than a tenfold increase in annual cardiac mortality rate in men with coronary heart disease [11].

References

1 Silverman, M. E.; Silverman, B.D.: The diagnostic capabilities and limitations of the electrocardiogram; in Hurst, Update II: The heart. Bypass surgery for obstructive coronary disease, pp. 13–45 (McGraw-Hill, New York 1980).

2 Amsterdam, E. A.; Dressendorfer, R. H.; Mason, D. T.: Toward improved interpretation of the exercise test. Cardiology *66:* 236–240 (1980).

3 Berman, D. S.; Amsterdam, E.A.; Joye, J. A.; Glass, E.; Levene, D.; DeNardo, G. L.; Mason, D. T.: Thallium-201 stress myocardial scintigraphy: application in asymptomatic patients with positive exercise electrocardiograms. Am. J. Cardiol. *41:* 380 (1978).

4 Williams, D. O.; Most, A. S.: Clinical, angiographic and hemodynamic characteristics of patients with a strongly positive exercise test. Cardiology *66:* 240–248 (1980).

5 Goldman, S.; Tselos, S.; Cohn, K.: Marked depth of ST-segment depression during treadmill exercise testing: Indicator of severe coronary artery disease. Chest *69:* 729 (1976).

6 Weisburst, M. R.; Most, A.S.; Williams, D. O.: Significance of the negative exercise test in evaluation of patients with chest pain. Clin. Cardiol. *2:* 33 (1979).

7 McNeer, J. F.; Margolis, J. R.; Lee, K. L.; Kisslo, J. A.; Peter, R. H.; Kong, Y.; Behar, V. S.; Wallace, A. G.; McCants, C. B.; Rosati, R. A.: The role of the exercise test in the evaluation of patients for ischemic heart disease. Circulation *57:* 71 (1978).

8 Robb, G. P.; Marks, H. H.: Postexercise electrocardiogram in arteriosclerotic heart disease. Its value in diagnosis and prognosis. J. Am. med. Ass. *200:* 918 (1967).

9 Bruschke, A. V. G.; Proudfit, W. L.; Sones, F. M.: Progress study of 590 consecutive nonsurgical cases of coronary disease followed 5–9 years. I. Arteriographic correlations. Circulation *47:* 1147 (1973).

10 Théroux, P.; Waters, D. D.; Halphen, C., et al.: Prognostic value of exercise testing soon after myocardial infarction. New Engl. J. Med. *301:* 341 (1979).

11 Bruce, R. A.; Peterson, D. R.; DeRouen, T., et al.: Noninvasive predictors of sudden cardiac death in men with coronary heart disease. Am. J. Cardiol. *39:* 833 (1977).

Prof. E. A. Amsterdam, MD, Chief, Coronary Care Unit, School of Medicine, University of California, Davis, CA 95616 (USA)

Adv. Cardiol., vol. 31, pp. 23–27 (Karger, Basel 1982)

Determination of Prognosis in Patients with Coronary Artery Disease by Noninvasive Radionuclide-Based Methods Applied during Exercise

J. S. Borer[1], P. Phillips, J. W. Moses, H. L. Goldberg[2], J. Fisher

Cardiology Division, New York Hospital-Cornell Medical Center, New York, N. Y., USA

Radionuclide-based methods have been found to be of great value in the diagnosis of coronary artery disease [1–3, 7, 11, 12]. Both thallium-based myocardial perfusion scintigraphy and technetium-based redionuclide cineangiography have been found to manifest diagnostic sensitivity and specificity in excess of 90 %. Since diagnosis with both methods is based on the detection of objective manifestations of ischemia induced by the interposition of physical stress, it is reasonable to infer that the severity of ischemia developed during stress also can be determined from these diagnostic studies. Moreover, it is reasonable to hypothesize that prognosis must in some way be directly related to the severity of ischemia, an inference which is consistent with experimental data regarding acute ischemic events [4].

During the past 2 years, several groups have collected data which, while preliminary, support the use of radionuclide-based methods in the determination of prognosis in patients with coronary artery disease. In fact, these data, in aggregate, suggest that the functional assessment of myocardial ischemia with radionuclide-based testing may importantly modify prognostic conclusions based on anatomic assessment of coronary stenoses by coronary arteriography.

Though myocardial perfusion scintigraphy with thallium-201 inherently is, at best, a semiquantitative technique in the assessment of myocardial ischemia, the direct visual evaluation of the extent of malperfu-

[1] J. S. B. is an Established Investigator of the American Heart Association.

[2] H. L. G. is the Isadore Rosenfeld Heart Foundation Fellow of New York Hospital-Cornell Medical Center.

sion now has been demonstrated to be of major prognostic value. In a retrospective study involving 138 patients who underwent coronary arteriography but did not receive coronary bypass grafting therapy, *Brown* et al. [5] compared results of thallium scintigraphy, contrast left ventriculography at rest and coronary arteriography as predictors of infarction or death during an average 3.7-year follow-up period. Myocardial images were obtained in two views both immediately after exercise and 2–4 h later and each view was divided into six segments. Analysis of these images indicated that, for the 100 patients without known previous myocardial infarctions, the number of transient (immediate postexercise only) scintigraphic perfusion defects was the only significant independent predictor of cardiac events. The number of diseased coronary arteries was independently predictive only when thallium data were not considered. For the 38 patients with known prior infarctions, left-ventricular ejection fraction at rest was the only significant independent predictor, but if ejection fraction was not considered, then the number of persistent (exercise and reperfusion) scintigraphic defects, together with thallium lung activity, were significantly predictive of the subsequent clinical course.

Jones [6] similarly found that ejection fraction at rest, in this case determined by first-pass radionuclide angiopraphy, was useful in identifying a group of patients with poor long-term prognosis. This finding was not unexpected in view of the similar results of multiple contrast-angiographic studies in the past. However, *Jones* [6] results represent an important addition to the contrast-angiographic studies because the radionuclide-based study involved patients who clinically were not necessarily sufficiently ill to require cardiac catheterization, the modality employed to obtain the earlier data. Moreover, *Jones'* [6] work further indicated the prognostic importance of exercise-induced abnormalities in left-ventricular function. Among 882 patients with clinically apparent ischemic heart disease and cardiac-catheterization-documented coronary stenoses who also underwent radionuclide angiography during exercise, 236 responded with an increase in ejection fraction during exercise. During an average 23-month follow-up, only 1 (0.004%) died. Of the 646 patients whose ejection fraction fell during exercise, 33 (5%) died. These data were mirrored in the results recorded among the 490 patients with clinical evidence of ischemic heart disease who did not undergo catheterization: of the 215 whose ejection fraction increased, none died during an average 31 months follow-up, while cardiac deaths occurred in 7 of the 275 (3%) whose ejection fraction fell. Moreover, paralleling the findings of *Brown* et al. [5], *Jones* [6] found that the number and location of coronary artery lesions was less predictive of 2-year natural history than was ejection fraction response: patients with three-vessel or moderate left main coronary stenoses were free of major events if exercise-induced ischemia was not apparent by radionuclide angiography, while patients with anatomically less severe abnormalities but with functional evidence of ischemia manifested a demonstrably higher mortality risk.

Attempts at more precise definition of prognosis based on radionuclide cineangiographic results currently are underway in our laboratory. However, while long-term epidemiologic studies are being performed, we have attempted to provide clinically useful insights into prognosis by determining the extent to which radionuclide cineangiographic results can predict the presence of other proven indicators of relatively high short-term risk. Thus, our initial attempt has been to define the relationship between radionuclide cineangiographic results and angiographic evidence of severe (≥ 75% luminal diameter obstruction) left main or severe proximal three-vessel coronary stenoses. Our preliminary results indicate that radionuclide cineangiography can predict the presence of such high-risk anatomical abnormalities with relatively high accuracy [9]. Thus, among 250 patients with angiographically demonstrable coronary artery disease and relatively mild symptoms, 10% manifested severe left main coronary stenosis and 18% manifested severe proximal stenosis of the three major arteries. When radionuclide cineangiography was performed, approximately one-third of the population had either an increase in ejection fraction during exercise or a minimal decrease (< 5%, the limits of reproducibility of the method); none of these patients had severe left main disease, and only a small number, all with a fall in ejection fraction during exercise, had proximal three-vessel disease [9]. Slightly more than a third of the population had a marked fall (≥ 10%) in ejection fraction during exercise, but the overwhelming majority of those with critical stenoses were in this group. Moreover, more than half of those patients with a ≥ 10% fall in ejection fraction during exercise manifested either severe left main or severe proximal three-vessel disease [9]. In addition, preliminary results from corollary studies indicate that the majority of those with severe ischemia during exercise who did not manifest severe left main or severe proximal three-vessel stenoses instead manifested moderate (50–74% reduction in luminal diameter) left main stenoses [10] or severe proximal stenosis of the left anterior descending coronary artery, often with no other or only one other coronary lesion [8]. Patients with these anatomical abnormalitites also are known to be at relatively higher risk than other arteriographically defined subgroups of patients. Thus, our preliminary results indicate that radionuclide cineangiography can be used to select patients with anatomical indicators of poor prognosis, and are consistent with the concept that the noninvasive functional assessment of ischemia severity by radionuclide cineangiography can provide valuable prognostic information in the patients with coronary artery disease.

References

1 Borer, J. S.; Bacharach, S. L.; Green, M. V.; Kent, K. M.; Epstein, S. E.; Johnston, G. S.: Real-time radionuclide cineangiography in the non-invasive evaluation of global and regional left ventricular function at rest and during exercise in patients with coronary artery disease. New Engl. J. Med. *296:* 839–844 (1977).
2 Borer, J. S.; Bacharach, S. L.; Green, M. V.; Kent, K. M.; Johnston, G. S.; Epstein, S. E.: Effect of nitroglycerin on exercise-induced abnormalities of left ventricular regional function and ejection fraction in coronary artery disease: assessment by radionuclide cineangiography in symptomatic and asymptomatic patients. Circulation *57:* 314–320 (1978).
3 Borer, J. S.; Kent, K. M.; Bacharach, S. L.; Green, M. V.; Johnston, G. S.; Epstein, S. E.: Sensitivity, specificity, and predictive accuracy of radionuclide cineangiography during exercise in patients with coronary artery disease. Circulation *60:* 572–580 (1979).
4 Borer, J. S.; Kent, K. M.; Goldstein, R. E.; Epstein, S. E.: Nitroglycerin-induced reduction in incidence of spontaneous ventricular fibrillation during coronary occlusion in dogs. Am. J. Cardiol. *33:* 517–520 (1974).
5 Brown, K. A.; Boucher, C. A.; Okada, R. D.; Newell, J.; Strauss, H. W.; Pohost, G. M.: The prognostic value of serial exercise thallium-201 imaging in patients presenting for evaluation of chest pain: comparison to contrast angiography, exercise electrocardiography, and clinical data (Abstract). Am. J. Cardiol. *49:* 967 (1982).
6 Jones, R. H.: Personal communication.
7 Jones, R. H.; Rerych, S. K.; Newman, G. E.; Scholz, P. M.; Howe, R.; Oldham, N.; Goodrich, J. K.; Sabiston, D. C.: Noninvasive radionuclide procedures for diagnosis and management of myocardial ischemia. Wld J. Surg. *2:* 811–828 (1978).
8 Phillips, P.; Borer, J. S.; Goldstein, J.; Jacobstein, J.; Moses, J.; Fisher, J.: Proximal left anterior descending coronary stenosis: the functional equivalent of triple vessel disease? (Abstract). Am. J. Cardiol. *49:* 957 (1982).
9 Phillips, P.; Borer, J. S.; Jacobstein, J.; Plancher, K.; Carter, J.; Moses, J.; Goldstein, J.; Collins, M.; Fisher, J.: Prognostically critical coronary stenoses: identification by radionuclide cineangiography (Abstract). Am. J. Cardiol. *49:* 991 (1982).
10 Phillips, P.; Borer, J. S.; Jacobstein, J.; Moses, J.; Goldstein, J. E.; Kligfield, P.; Collins, M.; Plancher, K.: Comparative sensitivity of exercise ECG and RNCA in detecting left main disease (Abstract). Clin. Res. *29:* 685A (1981).

11 Okada, R. D.; Boucher, C. A.; Kirshenbaum, H. K.; Kushner, F. G.; Strauss, H. W.; Block, P. C.; McKusick, K. A.; Pohost, G. M.: Improved diagnostic accuracy of thallium-201 stress test using multiple observers and criteria derived from interobserver analysis of variance. Am. J. Cardiol. *46:* 619–624 (1980).
12 Strauss, H. W.; Harrison, K.; Pitt, B.: Thallium-201: non-invasive determination of the regional distribution of cardiac output. J. nucl. Med. *18:* 1167–1170 (1977).

Jeffrey S. Borer, MD, New York Hospital-Cornell Medical Center,
525 East 68th Street, New York, NY 10021 (USA)

Adv. Cardiol., vol. 31, pp. 28–34 (Karger, Basel 1982)

Prognostic Value of Exercise Testing in Respect to Effects of Aortocoronary Bypass Surgery on Functional Aerobic Capacity

M. Niederberger, G. Gaul, W. Schlick, E. Wolner

Kardiologische Universitäts-Klinik (Vorstand: Prof. Dr. *F. Kaindl*), und II. Chirurgische Universitäts-Klinik (Vorstand: Prof. Dr. *E. Wolner*), Wien, Österreich

Introduction

It has been suggested that aortocoronary bypass grafting is indicated in symptomatic patients with coronary artery disease and ischemia who have the following: (1) disabling angina pectoris unresponsive to adequate medical management whether myocardial infarction has occurred or not; (2) critical stenosis of the left main coronary artery, or (3) triple vessel disease with moderate impairment of ventricular function [1]. However, the relative importance of anatomic and functional criteria has not been established [2].

It is conceivable that not the angiographically demonstrated severity of coronary arterial lesions but rather the functional reserve of the left ventricle is the most important determinant of survival [3]. Furthermore, patients with severe coronary artery disease but with little preoperative impairment of functional capacity may be relieved from chest pain at exertion but their exercise capacity may still be limited by other symptoms such as shortness of breath and the return to work may not be enhanced [4]. In order to investigate the functional effects of aortocoronary bypass grafting (ACBG) in relation to preoperative exercise tolerance, we analyzed two groups of patients whose pre- and postoperative cardiac evaluation was done at 2 independent hospitals in Vienna but who were all operated at the same department of surgery.

Table I. Group H (n = 51,)

a Supine bicycle exercise

Subgroup A $Watts_{SL_{max}}$ > 100, n = 24
Subgroup B $Watts_{SL_{max}}$ ≤ 100, n = 27
SL_{max} at symptom-limited maximal exercise.

b History of myocardial infarction	A	B
Anterior	4	8
Inferior/posterior	8	6
None	12	13

Table II. Comparison of subgroups A and B

	A	B
Age, years	53 ± 5	55 ± 7
Exercise capacity, %	80 ± 13	45 ± 10
SBP_{max}, mm Hg	219 ± 29	179 ± 24
$PAMP_{max}$, mm Hg	47 ± 9	44 ± 10
$PADP_{max}$, mm Hg	37 ± 7	33 ± 9
EF, %	64 ± 12	60 ± 15

Exercise capacity = % of sex- and age-adjusted normal values; SBP = systolic blood pressure; PAMP, PADP = pulmonary arterial mean, diastolic pressure; EF = left ventricular ejection fraction.

Subjects and Methods

51 men (group H) who were patients of hospital H had ACBG in 1980. Before and 1 month after ACBG, symptom-limited maximal bicycle exercise testing was performed in the supine position. The initial workload was 25 W and power was increased by 25 W every 2 min. Pulmonary arterial pressures were recorded by use of an indwelling microcatheter [5]. Retrospectively, the group was divided into subgroups A and B according to the patients preoperative exercise capacity (table I). Subgroups A and B did not differ in terms of age, pulmonary arterial pressures during supine bicycle exercise or left ventricular ejection fraction at rest, but together with lower exercise capacity the maximal systolic blood pressure was also less in subgroup B (table II). The coronary score, the number of highly stenotic vessels and the

Table III. Comparison of subgroups A and B

	A	B
Coronary score	42 ± 14	41 ± 16
>70% stenotic vessels (n)	2.5 ± 0.7	2.5 ± 0.8
Bypass grafts (n)	2.4 ± 0.7	2.2 ± 0.8
Perioperative infarctions (n)	4/24	1/27

Table IV. Group K (n = 58; 56 ♂, 2 ♀)

I (n = 15):	Exercise capacity ≥ 50% *and* SBP_{max} ≥ 160 mm Hg
II, III:	Exercise capacity < 50% *or* SBP_{max} < 160 mm Hg
	II (n = 24): LVEDP < 16 mm Hg *and* EF ≥ 50%
	III (n = 19): LVEDP ≥ 16 mm Hg *or* EF < 50%

Table V. Comparison of subgroups I, II and III

	I	II	III
Age, years	52 ± 5	50 ± 7	54 ± 5
Exercise capacity, %	68 ± 14	42 ± 19	32 ± 19
SBP_{max}, mm Hg	193 ± 30	161 ± 22	164 ± 32
LVEDP, mm Hg	16 ± 6	14 ± 4	23 ± 6
EF, %	70 ± 14	69 ± 11	51 ± 16

Exercise capacity = % of sex- und age-adjusted normal values; SBP = systolic blood pressure; LVEDP = left ventricular end-diastolic pressure at rest; EF = left ventricular ejection at rest.

Table VI. Comparison of subgroups I, II and III

		I	II	III
>70% stenotic vessels (n)		2.47 ± 0.8	2.46 ± 0.8	2.53 ± 0.8
Bypass grafts (n)		1.93 ± 0.6	2.00 ± 0.8	2.28 ± 0.8
Nitro	pre./postop. (n)	10/7	21/13	17/12
Beta-blockers	pre./postop. (n)	9/4	9/3	7/5
Digitalis	pre./postop. (n)	3/5	8/12	6/10

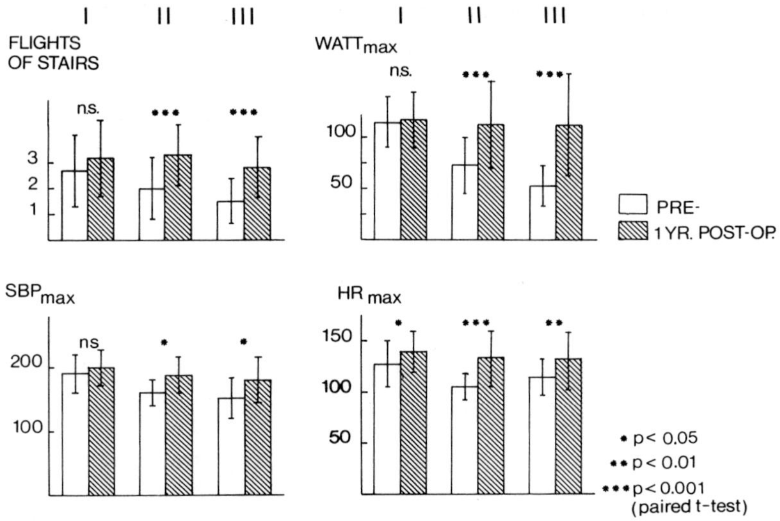

Fig. 1. Effects of ACBG on exercise tolerance (n = 51).

number of bypass grafts were similar in both subgroups but, perioperatively, more acute myocardial infarctions were observed in subgroup A (table III).

56 men and 2 women (group K) who were patients of hospital C had ACBG before 1980. Symptom-limited maximal bicycle exercise testing was performed in the upright position before and 1 year after surgery. The initial workload was 25 W and power was increased by 25 W every 2 min [6]. Retrospectively, the group was subdivided into 3 subgroups according to preoperative results from exercise testing and indices of left ventricular function at rest (table IV). The subgroups did not differ in respect to age (table V) and number of highly stenotic coronary vessels or of bypass grafts (table VI).

Results

The results of group H are shown in figure 1. In comparison with preoperative values, exercise capacity was reduced 1 month postoperatively in subgroup A but was increased in subgroup B. Systolic blood pressures and heart rates at symptom limited maximal exercise (SBP_{max}, HR_{max}) were higher postoperatively only in subgroup B, whereas ST segment depression as well as pulmonary arterial mean ($PAMP_{max}$) and diastolic pressure ($PADP_{max}$) at symptom-limited exercise were reduced postoperatively in both subgroups.

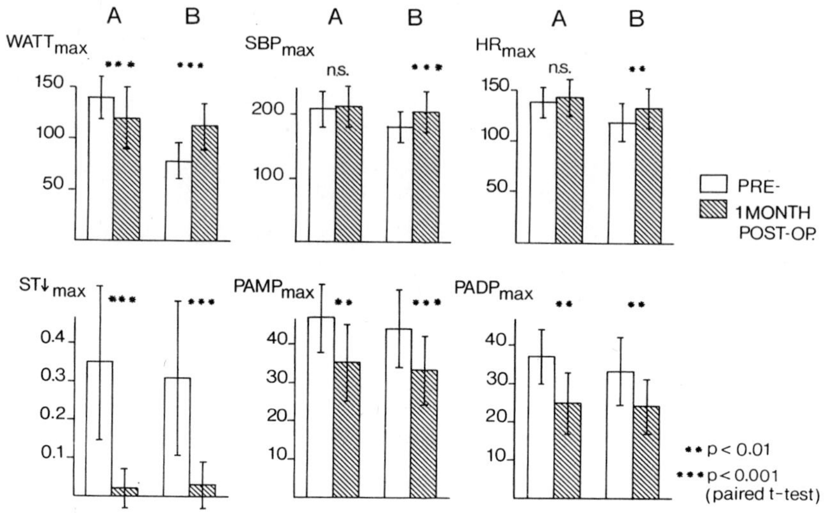

Fig. 2. Effects of ACBG on exercise tolerance (n = 58).

The results of group K are shown in figure 2. 1 year after ACBG, exercise capacity as defined by the ability of climbing stairs or by bicycle ergometry and systolic blood pressure at symptom-limited maximal bicycle exercise were increased only in subgroups II and III. All subgroups demonstrated higher heart rate at symptom-limited maximal bicycle exercise postoperatively.

Discussion

Our results indicate that measurements from exercise testing are important prognostic indices in respect to the effect of ACBG on exercise tolerance, independent of the severity of anatomic coronary lesions as demonstrated by coronary angiography. 1 month after surgery, the reduction of exercise capacity in patients with relatively little preoperative impairment of exercise tolerance despite severe coronary artery disease may be explained by a reduction of whole body performance due to deconditioning. The loss of exertional ST segment depressions in subgroups A and B after surgery and the reduction of pulmonary arterial pressures at symptom-limited exercise are in accordance with improvement of coronary blood flow and reduced myocardial ischemia. Obviously, exercise capacity was not primarily limited by angina pectoris but by other symptoms such as dyspnea or general fatigue.

However, even 1 year after ACBG, preoperatively less impaired patients did not demonstrate a measurable improvement of exercise capacity. On the other hand, preoperatively severely impaired patients whose exercise capacity was reduced below 50% of the sex- and age-adjusted normal values or whose blood pressure response during exercise was restricted, supposedly due to left ventricular dysfunction as a consequence of reversible myocardial ischemia, demonstrated functional improvement 1 year after ACBG, independent of preoperative indices of left ventricular dysfunction at rest.

These results may be related to the results of other studies which demonstrate the prognostic importance of preoperative exercise capacity in respect to survival with medical treatment. From a series of 100 inoperable patients with severe coronary lesions, it was concluded that exercise capacity is a nonspecific but very sensitive predictor of good prognosis in coronary heart disease [7]. In patients with relatively little functional impairment the mortality rate is low also after myocardial infarction [8–11].

Therefore, in patients with coronary heart disease, whether with a history of myocardial infarction or not and independent of left ventricular function at rest as well as of angiographically documented coronary anatomy, exercise capacity and measurements from exercise testing such as the systolic blood pressure response can serve as prognostic indices for survival without surgery and for functional improvement by aortocoronary bypass grafting.

References

1 Council Report: Indications for aortocoronary bypass graft surgery. J. Am. med. Ass. *242:* 2709 (1979).

2 Mcintosh, H. D.; Buccino, R. A.: Is bypass grafting indicated for all patients with atherosclerosis of the left main coronary artery? Am. J. Cardiol. *45:* 521–523 (1980).

3 Bruce, R. A.; DeRouen, T. A.; Hammermeister, K. E.: Noninvasive screening criteria for enhanced 4-year survival after aortocoronary bypass surgery. Circulation *60:* 638–646 (1979).

4 Hammermeister, K. E.; DeRouen, T. A.; English, M. T.; Dodge, H. T.: Effect of surgical versus medical therapy on return to work in patients with coronary artery disease. Am. J. Cardiol. *44:* 105–111 (1979).

5 Kubicek, F.; Gaul, G.: Comparison of supine and sitting body position during a triangular exercise test. Eur. J. appl. Physiol. *36:* 275–285 (1977).
6 Niederberger, M.; Kubicek, F.; Reiterer, W.: Leitlinien für die Ergometrie. Acta. med. austriaca *2:* 33 (1975).
7 Broustet, J. P.; Coue, J. C.; Pic, A.; Saliou, B.; Guern, P.: Predictive value of symptom-limited exercise testing for life expectancy in inoperable coronary patients with disabling angina. Cardiology *68:* suppl. 2 (1981).
8 Velasco, J. A.; Tormo, V.; Ridocci, F.; Blanch, S.: Early load-limited versus symptom-limited exercise testing. Prognostic value in 206 myocardial infarction patients. Cardiology *68:* suppl. 2 (1981).
9 DeBacker, G. G.; Weyne, T.; Derese, A.: Prognostic value of exercise tresting. A 6-year follow-up in post-myocardial infarction patients. Cardiology *68:* suppl. 2 (1981).
10 Samek, L.; Greene, R.; Droste, C.; Betz, P.; Roskamm, H.: Results of exercise tests and prognosis in postinfarction patients below age 40. Cardiology *68:* suppl. 2 (1981).
11 Hayet, M.; Kellermann, J. J.: The angina pectoris threshold heart rate as a prognostic sign, results of a 5-year follow-up. Cardiology *68:* suppl. 2 (1981).

Doz. Dr. M. Niederberger, Kardiologische Universitätsklinik,
Garnisonsgasse 13, A-1090 Wien (Austria)

Adv. Cardiol., vol. 31, pp. 35–37 (Karger, Basel 1982)

Systolic Time Intervals: Prognostic Value and Exercise Responses

David H. Spodick

University of Massachusetts Medical School and Division of Cardiology, St. Vincent Hospital, Worcester, Mass., USA

Systolic time intervals (STIs) are a paradigm of truly noninvasive, infinitely repeatable, inexpensive and precise methodology. They respond to physiologic, pathologic and pharmacologic interventions that stimulate or block the adrenergic and cholinergic nervous systems and those that alter contractility, preload and afterload.

In primary myocardial diseases, in myocardial abnormalities associated with valve and coronary disease and in pericardial and endocardial diseases STIs reflect abnormal function. In patients with wall motion abnormalities, they are often more reliable than M-mode echocardiographic measurements.

During *exercise* – upright and supine, treadmill and bicycle, dynamic and isometric – and in recovery, changes in STIs reflect the physiologic responses obtained by invasive testing and are more suitable for beat-to-beat measurements. In patients with heart disease these responses can yield diagnostic results. For *cardiocirculatory challenges* such as tilt and Valsalva maneuver, comparable physiologic and pathologic responses can be obtained.

STIs are particularly reliable for monitoring pharmacologic responses, notably to digitalis glycosides, sympathomimetic agents, nitrates and β-adrenoceptor-blocking agents.

A readily understood example of how systolic time intervals change without intervention is *pulsus alternans*. In this circumstance, alternating beats originating from the same pacemaker and at virtually identical cycle lengths show alternating function, so that there are continuing pairs of weak and strong beats. In strong beats the preejection period (PEP) is shorter and lengthens in weak beats; this is mainly due to changes in isovolumic contraction time. Strong beats are also characterized by longer left-ventricular ejection time (and hence ejection time index, ETI) so that the net expression of cardiac function, PEP/LVET, represents these reciprocal changes in its numerator and denominator even more strongly, i.e. PEP/LVET is much smaller in strong beats.

In 277 ambulatory subjects investigated every 2 years, there were 112 with *ischemic heart disease* and 165 normal control subjects. STIs were significantly different between the groups: for ischemic heart disease versus controls ETI = 356 versus 366 ms; PEP = 107 versus 99 ms; PEP/LVET 0.41 versus 0.36; pulse transmission time 20 versus 24 ms (p values = 0.001 for all, except PEP/LVET < 0.05). Among 11 patients with *congestive cardiomyopathy* matched for sex and age with 11 patients with *coronary heart disease,* differences in PEP, PEP/LVET, ETI and pulse transmission time (PTT) were all significant, i.e. $p < 0.05 - < 0.001$. Thus, PEP was much longer, ETI shorter and PEP/LVET much larger in the patients with cardiomyopathy. The latter also had a 50% longer PTT (32.9 versus 22.5 ms).

When patients with *chest pain* were divided between those with no anatomic coronary disease and one-, two-, and three-vessel disease the PEP showed a stepwise increase from no anatomic disease to three-vessel disease. The PEP/LVET showed a comparable difference, with differences significant for every disease level between groups. The ETI, however, did not show consistent differences, although the smallest level was in three-vessel disease (differing from those with no anatomic disease at $p < 0.02$). In patients with *acute myocardial infarct* followed with daily STI, *Northover* showed the mean level of PEP/LVET to be consistently higher in nonsurvivors than in survivors. In patients with *angina,* life table analysis for 5-year survival utilizing the PEP/LVET cutpoint of 0.5 by *Gillilan* demonstrated that those with PEP/LVET less than 0.50 had approximately 90% survival whereas those over 0.50 had under 10% survival. The most striking differences appeared between 6 months and 2.5 years because of a precipitous drop in survival in the latter group.

STIs have been successfully applied to *exercise* studied by the development of the *ear densitograph* which permits a steady trace during movement so that STI during exercise performance as well as before and after could be accurately monitored. These show changes in PEP (decrease) and ETI (increase) as well as PEP/LVET (decrease) entirely consistent with the known physiology of exercise, i.e. vagal withdrawal followed by sympathetic stimulation, accompanied by variably increased stroke volume and increased ejection rate. Normal subjects further show rapid restitution at the end of exercise.

In patients who have had coronary angiograms, changes in the PEP and PEP/LVET were highly sensitive to the presence of significant disease during treadmill exercise (Bruce Protocol). When PEP/LVET was calculated as change from rest to exercise, the changes at 1 min and 4 min showed clear separation of angiogram-negative and angiogram-positive subjects. When a comparable group with angiography but taking a beta-adrenergic blocking agent was comparably exercised, the clear division of change in PEP/LVET was no longer found, although there were still some differences between groups: the change due to treatment with beta-adrenergic blockade nearly normalized the response in those with abnormal arteriograms.

Recently, ear densitography has been adapted to ambulatory monitoring by feeding the output of the densitograph into one channel of a two-channel Holter monitor. Initial results with volunteer subjects have been promising in that STIs follow each level of activity. However, a larger series is needed for a conclusive evaluation in subjects with heart disease.

Prof. D. H. Spodick, MD, Division of Cardiology, University of Massachusetts, St. Vincent Hospital, Worcester, MA 01110 (USA)

Adv. Cardiol., vol. 31, pp. 38–44 (Karger, Basel 1982)

Prognostic Significance of Exercise-Induced Ventricular Arrhythmias in Postmyocardial Infarction Patients

G. De Backer

Department of Cardiology, Akademisch Ziekenhuis, Gent, Belgium

The prognostic and clinical significance of exercise-related ventricular premature beats (VPB) has been controversial in cardiology for many years. Numerous investigators have believed and demonstrated that exercise-induced ventricular arrhythmias are an abnormal finding while others believe that it is of no significance. However, when the published reports are compared, the composition of the patient groups is found to vary tremendously. Numerous studies deal with referrals for the evaluation of chest pain. This selection can result in a large difference in the extent of coronary heart disease between study populations depending on local referral rules and habits. It has been shown that ventricular arrhythmias tend to correlate with the extent of the coronary lesions as well as with the presence of wall motion abnormalities. So, when two study groups that differ substantially in prevalence of coronary heart disease are compared, it should not be a surprise that the prevalence of VPBs as well as their prognostic significance are found to be different. In order to avoid this heterogeneity in the study population, the question of the prognostic significance of exercise-related VPB as discussed in this paper is limited to groups of patients who have developed a documented myocardial infarct.

In most rehabilitation centers symptom-limited maximal exercise testing is used in postinfarct patients between the 4th and the 12th weeks after the infarct. The prevalence of exercise-induced ventricular ectopy in such patients varies from 35 to 70%, averaging 50%. It should be emphasized that a continuous recording system improves the detection rate of VPBs during exercise. Especially the disclosure of complex and repetitive forms of VPBs is enhanced by continuous systems. *Fitzgerald* et al. [1] have demonstrated that the prevalence of exercise-induced ventricular

Table I. Prognostic significance of exercise-induced VPB in postinfarct patients tested at ± 10 weeks

	Granath et al. [2]	*De Backer* et al. [3]	*DeBusk* et al. [4]	*De Backer* et al. [5]
Patients, n	174	302	80	112
Mean age, years	59	52	52	52
Test period, weeks	9	10	11	10
Maximal heart rate/min	126	143	145	144
Mean follow-up period, years	2.5	3	2	6
Exercise-induced VPB				
Prevalence, %				
Any	–	57	53	54
Complex	23	17	30	30
Prognostic significance	yes	no	no	no

ectopy is stable from the 3rd to the 12th month after the infarct; this means that when the prevalence rate of ventricular ectopy is compared at 3, 6 or 9 months after the infarct, no significant differences are observed, the rate averaging 50%.

In table I the findings observed in four different studies are summarized [2–5]. In all four studies the tests were performed around the 10th week after the infarct. In three studies the mean age was 52 years while in the Swedish study the patients were somewhat older. The maximal heart rate achieved was lower in the Swedish study because of a stop condition at a heart rate of 140/min, while in the three other studies the test was symptom-limited. The prevalence of exercise-induced VPBs varied from 53 to 57% while complex VPBs, defined by frequent or multifocal or pairs or runs of VPB, were found in 17–30%. The prognostic significance was studied over a period varying from 2 to 6 years. In three studies no prognostic significance was observed while in the Swedish study a mortality of 40% was observed in those with complex ventricular arrhythmias during the exercise test as compared to 19% in those without arrhythmias.

In table II more details are given on two of our own studies [3, 5]. One of the studies included 112 patients and was completed after a 6-year follow-up in all subjects. In the other study the follow-up period varies and averages 3 years. The incidence of cardiovascular events was defined by cardiovascular mortality and nonfatal recurrent infarct.

Table II. Prognostic significance of exercise-induced VPB in postinfarct patients tested at 10 weeks

	De Backer et al. [3] (n = 302)	*De Backer* et al. [5] (n = 112)
Incidence of cardiovascular events, %	11/3 years	36/6 years
Prevalence of VPB		
Any VPB, %	57	55
Pairs or runs, %	17	30
Prognostic significance		
Any VPB		
Sensitivity, %	59	53
Predictive value, %	12	34
Pairs or runs		
Sensitivity, %	6	25
Predictive value, %	4	29

The prognostic significance of exercise-induced ventricular ectopy is presented as sensitivity and predictive value figures. Sensitivity is the ratio of patients presenting with cardiovascular events and ventricular ectopy to the total number of patients presenting with cardiovascular events. So, 53 and 59% of all those presenting with new cardiovascular events had developed VPBs during the exercise test as compared to 55 and 57% in the total groups. 25 and 6% of all those presenting with new cardiovascular events had developed either pairs or runs of VPBs during the exercise test as compared to 30 and 17% in the total groups. The predictive value is the ratio of patients presenting with cardiovascular events and ventricular ectopy to the total number of patients presenting ventricular ectopy. So, from all those who presented with VPBs during the exercise test 34% and 12% developed a new cardiovascular event as compared to 36 and 11% in the total group. From all those with pairs or runs of VPBs during the exercise test 29 and 4% developed a new cardiovascular event as compared to 36 and 11% in the total group. When statistical tests are applied to these figures, the only significant finding is that the incidence of new events was significantly lower in the group with pairs or runs of VPBs during exercise as compared to the others in the study on 302 subjects.

During more recent years exercise testing before discharge from hospital in postinfarct patients has become widespread for a variety of reasons. The safety of such a procedure has been demonstrated. Again the question can be asked about the clinical and prognostic significance of

Table III. Prognostic significance of exercise-induced VPB in postinfarct patients tested before hospital discharge

Reference	Patients n	Age years	Test period days	Exercise test method	Follow-up period years	Exercise-induced VPB		
						prevalence		Prognostic significance
						any	complex	
2	205	59	21	submaximal	2.5	?	17	yes
6	62	60	18	submaximal	1.7	21	?	no
7	210	53	11	submaximal	1	20	4	no [1]
8	166	?	14	submaximal	1.6	?	?	no
9	195	54	21	submaximal + symptom-limited maximal	2	38	?	no
10	236	57	16	submaximal	1	43	22	yes
11	317	?	18	symptom-limited maximal	5.7	?	15	yes
12	200	52	21	submaximal	3	?	3	no

[1] Yes for sudden death.

ventricular ectopy induced by such a test before discharge. In table III results are summarized from some of these studies [2, 6–12]. The mean age of the study groups varies from 50 to 60 years. The test was performed from the 11th to the 21st days after the infarct. All authors used a submaximal test design except for two who used a symptom-limited maximal test. The follow-up period varies but exceeds 1 year in all studies. The prognostic significance in predicting new cardiovascular events and especially cardiovascular mortality was demonstrated in three studies and not observed in five, although one of these found an excess of sudden deaths among subjects with exercise-induced VPBs.

In table IV these results are related to some other findings observed in these studies. The percentage of subjects with clinical signs of heart failure at the time of the test is presented as well as the percentage of those on digitalis therapy at the time of the test. Furthermore the 1-year cardiovascular mortality and the prognostic significance of exercise-induced ventricular ectopy is presented.

In those studies where exercise-induced ventricular ectopy was found to be of prognostic significance, the percentage of patients with either signs

Table IV. Prognostic significance of exercise-induced VPB in postinfarct patients tested before hospital discharge

Reference	Heart failure %	Digitalis therapy %	1-year cardio-vascular mortality %	Exercise-induced VPB, prognostic significance
2	66	66	±15	yes
6	?	?	?	no
7	none	10	9	no [1]
8	?	?	?	no
9	none	none	< 2	no
10	41	41	12	yes
11	?	20	±15	yes
12	?	10	4	no

[1] Yes for sudden death.

of heart failure or on digitalis therapy is high. In those studies where no significant prognostic value was observed for the exercise-induced VPBs, no data on heart failure or digitalis therapy are available or the available data are markedly lower. *Davidson* et al. [9] excluded patients on digitalis therapy or with clinical signs of heart failure. In contrast to the study of *Granath* et al. [2], two thirds of all patients were on digitalis therapy because of clinical signs of heart failure. The 1-year cardiovascular mortality in the groups with a low percentage of patients with heart failure is also low: 4% in the study of *Velasco* et al. [12] and less than 2% in the study of *Davidson and DeBusk* [9]. On the contrary, it averages 15% in the studies of *Granath* et al. [2] and *Saunamäki and Damgaard Andersen* [11], where 66 and 20% of the patients were on digitalis therapy. In those studies with a high percentage of patients with heart failure or on digitalis, and a high 1-year cardiovascular mortality, the prognostic value of exercise-induced ventricular ectopy is also significant. This does not mean that the prognostic significance of exercise-induced ventricular ectopy as found in some of these studies is entirely explicable through the interrelation with left ventricular dysfunction, but clinical signs of heart failure and/or digitalis therapy are clearly confounding variables that must be considered in the analysis. *Weld* et al. [10] and *Saunamäki and Damgaard Andersen* [11] have tried to separate both ventricular function and arrhythmias and conclude that exercise-induced ventricular ectopy is of prognostic significance independent of left ventricular dysfunction.

So, the data available today on the clinical and prognostic significance of exercise-induced ventricular arrhythmias in post infarct patients are still controversial. The majority of studies has shown that exercise-induced ventricular ectopy by itself is not very valuable in predicting new events in postinfarct patients. The fact that approximately 50% of all postinfarct patients manifest some forms of ventricular ectopy with exercise by itself reduces the importance of the issue of the significance or the predictive value of this finding in the individual patient.

However, some features of the arrhythmias may provide insight in to a few other aspects of the postinfarct management. It has been suggested that certain forms of exercise-induced ventricular ectopy may be useful in identifying patients with significant two- or three-vessel disease, although others did not confirm this finding. The relation between exercise-induced ventricular ectopy and impaired left ventricular function reduces the prognostic significance of exercise-induced ventricular arrhythmias but allows to identify a subset of patients with a greater chance for such functional abnormalities. So, by combining various exercise-related variables it becomes possible to isolate from the postinfarct population a subset of low-risk patients, in whom a minimum of investigations is required, and a subset of high-risk patients, where a more aggressive management is clearly indicated. Exercise-induced ventricular arrhythmia in general or particular forms of it should further be studied in such multivariate predictive analysis, not only for their possible prognostic value but also because they provide useful tools in the decision-making rules for the optimal management of postinfarct patients.

References

1 Fitzgerald, J. W.; Houston, N.; DeBusk, R. F.: Natural history of ventricular arrhythmias in post-infarction patients. Circulation *54:* suppl. II, p. 10 (1976).

2 Granath, A.; Södermark, T.; Winge, T.; Volpe, U.; Zetterquist, S.: Early work load tests for evaluation of long-term prognosis of acute myocardial infarction. Br. Heart J. *39:* 758 (1977).

3 DeBacker, G.; Mercelis, L.; Durme, J. P. van; Verheye, S.; Egmond, J. van: The prognostic significance of an exercise test performed within three months after acute myocardial infarction; in Broustet, Bricaud, Denolin, Les épreuves d'effort, p. 203 (Expansion Scientifique Française, Paris 1978).

4 DeBusk, R. F.; Davidson, D. M.; Houston, N.; Fitzgerald, J.: Serial ambulatory electrocardiography and treadmill exercise testing after uncomplicated myocardial infarction. Am. J. Cardiol. *45:* 547 (1980).

5 De Backer, G.; Weyne, T.; Derese, T.: Prognostic significance of exercise testing: a 6-year follow-up in post-myocardial infarction patients. Cardiology *68:* suppl. 2, 71 (1981).

6 Smith, J. W.; Dennis, C. A.; Gasmann, A.; Gaines, J. A.; Staman, M.; Phibbs, B.; Marcus, F. I.: Exercise testing three weeks after myocardial infarction. Chest *75:* 12 (1979).

7 Theroux, P.; Waters, D. D.; Halphen, C.; Debaisieux, J. L.; Mizgala, H. F.: Prognostic value of exercise testing soon after myocardial infarction. New Engl. J. Med. *301:* 341 (1979).

8 Scardi, S.; Gori, P.; Pivotti, F.; Salvi, R.; Zibio, G.; Camerini, F.: Prognostic value of an early exercise test after acute myocardial infarction. Eur. Congr. Cardiology, 1980, Abstracts, vol. VIII, p. 86.

9 Davidson, D. M.; DeBusk, R. F.: Prognostic value of a single exercise test 3 weeks after uncomplicated myocardial infarction. Circulation *61:* 236 (1980).

10 Weld, F. M.; Chu, K. L.; Bigger, J. T.; Rolnitzky, L. M.: Risk stratification with low-level exercise testing 2 weeks after acute myocardial infarction. Circulation *64:* 306 (1981).

11 Saunamäki, K. I.; Damgaard Andersen, J.: Early exercise-test in the assessment of long-term prognosis after acute myocardial infarction. Acta med. scand. *209:* 185 (1981).

12 Valesco, J.; Tormo, V.; Ferrer, L. M.; Ridocci, F.; Blanck, S.: Early exercise test for evaluation of long-term prognosis after uncomplicated myocardial infarction. Eur. Heart J. *2:* 401 (1981).

G. De Backer, MD, Department of Cardiology, Akademisch Ziekenhuis, De Pintelaan 135, B-9000 Gent (Belgium)

Adv. Cardiol., vol. 31, pp. 45–50 (Karger, Basel 1982)

Indications for Coronary Bypass Surgery, 1982

Controlled Trials Scientifically and Ethically Optimum

David H. Spodick

University of Massachusetts Medical School and Division of Cardiology,
St. Vincent Hospital, Worcester, Mass., USA

The efficacy of any treatment depends on proof that it improves the patient's condition as compared to alternate treatment or no treatment. Conclusive proof demands appropriate standards of comparison, that is, that the patient would be dead or his condition worse without the therapeutic intervention. This is accomplished by an appropriate control group, i.e. (1) determined by methods which make control and treatment groups genuinely comparable in every significant respect, and (2) investigated concurrently. The scientific (hence, ethical) way to do this is by randomized prospective controlled trials [1–3].

Context

Indications for coronary artery bypass graft (CABG) at any time must be considered in its current context, i.e. the state of the art and state of the science of surgical and medical treatment of the condition. Thus, the following considerations are paramount in deciding the value of CABG:

(1) extremely low perioperative mortality associated with technically good surgery and anesthesia;

(2) long-term patency of vein and internal mammary artery grafts;

(3) excellent improvement of symptoms;

(4) better postoperative quality of life without necessarily returning to work;

(5) reduced subsequent hospitalization;

(6) deterioration from 2 to 10 years postoperatively in some patients;

(7) increased survival in certain high-risk subsets of patients (shown by

randomized controlled trials including the Veterans Administration Cooperative Study, and certain matched paired studies);

(8) newer antianginal and anti-coronary spasm agents deserving of further trial in comparison with CABG;

(9) no effect of CABG on *resting* left ventricular function (unless there is a mechanical cause);

(10) increased exercise tolerance, at least partly due to relief of pain;

(11) indications for postinfarction patients: (a) absence of Q waves implies higher risk, (b) indications essentially the same as without prior infarction but, when indicated, operation becomes more urgent;

(12) additional considerations: other diseases; patient's lifestyle and biologic age.

All studies agree that significant left main coronary disease, particularly in symptomatic patients, benefits from CABG which should be considered urgently as soon as left main coronary disease is demonstrated. As to *clinical predictors of statistical benefit,* the Veterans Administration randomized study showed that with or without left main coronary disease the following showed surgery to be beneficial [4]:

(1) ST depression on resting ECG;

(2) history of infarction;

(3) history of hypertension, and

(4) New York Heart Association functional class III, IV.

Clinical, anatomic and functional predictors (in the Seattle Heart Watch [5] matched-pair study showing surgery to be statistically beneficial) were: two- or three-vessel stenosis $\geq$ 70%; left main coronary disease; ejection fraction $\geq$ 30%; age $\geq$ 48 years, and absence of: murmurs, diuretic treatment or congestive heart failure, ventricular arrhythmia of any kind and cardiomegaly.

In postinfarction patients, *Sohn* et al. [6] predicted 5-year survival by *systolic time intervals.* PEP/LVET, when abnormal, predicted better survival in the surgical group; when normal ($\leq$ 0.42), there was no significant difference in survival, medical vs. surgical.

Chronic Stable Angina

Randomized studies in chronic stable angina show better surgical than medical survival in left main coronary disease and three-vessel disease subgroups, with strong indications that two-vessel disease may also be improved. This was particularly apparent in the high-risk tercile of the Veterans Administration Cooperative Study. The results of that randomized trial indicate that bypass is definitely better for 50% or greater stenosis of the left main coronary, for three-vessel disease with advanced stenosis of two vessels (especially the right and left anterior descending) and persistent pain or ischemia on medical treatment.

Congestive heart failure without mechanical complications may be aided if there is reversible ischemia and low ejection fraction. Congestive failure alone is not an indication for CABG without resection of aneurysm.

Selection for CABG in stable angina must consider severity of symptoms and response to exercise testing. Though most patients do not have a marked response, markedly positive exercise test (ST depression ≥ 2 mm, especially occurring early and lasting) implies a poor response to medical treatment and should lead to early angiography and consideration for CABG. Intermediate ST responses are not predictive of results of medical therapy.

Unstable Angina pectoris

Appropriately designed investigations show that careful medical management relieves unstable angina and that most such patients are not in a 'preinfarction' syndrome. The NHLBI randomized trial showed no advantage for surgery in considering *early* mortality or infarction so that early medical treatment is justified. *Pugh* et al. [7] showed total (in hospital plus follow-up) mortality to be comparable for medical and surgical patients, with all in-hospital infarcts in the surgical group, but severe angina during follow-up only in the medical group. In 1975, *Selden* et al. [8] first showed that intensive medical management could result in comparable prognosis but, again, severe angina during follow-up was almost entirely in the medical group. *Bertolasi* et al. [9] divided unstable angina into an *intermediate syndrome* and *progressive angina.* Patients with the intermediate syndrome had prolonged severe recurrent angina with transient ST and/or T wave changes with pain unrelated to exercise during the month prior to admission, plus absence of noncardiac disease, pump failure, prolonged arrhythmia and enzyme increases, and little or no response to nitrates. Prognostic results and severe angina during follow-up clearly favored the surgical group. The other group, progressive angina, was defined as a change in pain during 3 months without the criteria for the intermediate syndrome. Their mortality results did not favor either group, but severe angina during follow-up appeared only in the medical group. Summarizing the studies of *Pugh* et al. [7], *Selden* et al. [8] and *Bertolasi* et al. [9]: mortality during follow-up was between 0 and 25 % for the medical group and only 0–5 % in the surgical group. Infarcts occurred equally during follow-up in each (12 and 13 %, respectively). Severe angina varied from 17 to 63 % in the medical group and from 0 to 14 % in the surgical group. Thus, for unstable angina, intensive medical treatment with propranolol and nitrates and now, perhaps, the newer agents, is indicated to stabilize the patient, followed in a few days by angiography with the decision to operate individualized at that time.

Acute Myocardial Infarction

Initial studies appear to be favorable in this condition but they are not appropriately designed. Those conducting them, despite sometimes large numbers of patients, have called for appropriately designed, randomized, controlled studies but appear not to be planning to do them themselves.

Asymptomatic Patients with Positive Exercise Tests

Ambulatory monitoring has showed that up to 30 % of ST depressions were associated with angina. The remaining 70 % were symptom-free. Despite this, there is a poor correlation between a positive exercise test and coronary disease *in asymptomatic individuals.* Moreover, nitroglycerine given throughout the day decreases the frequency of even asymptomatic ST depression in ambulatory tracings. Because of the poor specificity of exercise ECG, these individuals should have radioisotope studies with exercise to evaluate any asymptomatic ST depressions. On the other hand, if the exercise ECG is positive at a low load and/or the ST depression is prolonged, coronary angiography should be performed to identify critical stenoses for possible CABG. Other studies may be added to determine whether coronary disease is present with *evidence of ischemia other than pain:* perfusion abnormality, abnormal regional contraction, elevated left-ventricular end-diastolic pressure or lactate production.

Symptomatic Coronary Spasm in the Presence of Atherosclerosis

These patients usually have chest pain and ST *elevation* (ST depression may also occur with spasm). Surgical results are not as good as in patients with effort angina who develop ST depressions. Treatment can be begun with vasodilators, with the subsequent decision to catheterize and treat individualized.

Patients Resuscitated from Sudden Cardiac Death

In the absence of infarction, resuscitated patients have an increased risk of further arrests, with high mortality in the first and second year after resuscitation. Evidence of ventricular arrhythmias refractory to treatment may call for myocardial resection, under which circumstances CABG may be added.

Indications for CABG 1982

Current indications aim for one or both of two objectives: relief of symptoms and improvement of prognosis.

Symptomatic Relief

Disabling angina refractory to medical therapy, symptomatic left main coronary disease, unstable angina with suitable vessels (two- or three-vessel disease; left main coronary disease) and variant angina with anatomic coronary disease.

Improvement of Prognosis

Left main coronary stenosis $\geq 50\%$, cardiogenic shock with suitable vessels (plus resection if necessary), three-vessel disease $\geq 50\%$ stenosis, ejection fraction $\geq 30\%$, two or three suitable vessels, (?) valve surgery with coronary stenoses and (?) asymptomatic patients with strongly positive exercise ECG/radionuclide tests.

References

1 Spodick, D. H.: Revascularization of the heart – Numerators in search of denominators (Editorial). Am. Heart J. *81:* 149–157 (1971).
2 Spodick, D. H.: The surgical mystique and the double standard: controlled trials of medical and surgical therapy for cardiac disease: analysis, hypothesis, proposal. Am. Heart J. *85:* 579–583 (1973).
3 Spodick, D. H.: Aortocoronary bypass surgery: emerging triumph of controlled clinical trials. Chest *71:* 318–319 (1977).

4 Detre, K.; Peduzzi, P.; Murphy, M.; et al.: Effect of bypass surgery on survival in patients in low- and high-risk subgroups delineated by the use of simple clinical variables. Circulation *63:* 1329–1338 (1981).
5 DeRouen, T. A.: Hammermeister, K. E.: Dodge, H. T.: Comparisons of the effects on survival after coronary artery surgery in subgroups of patients from the Seattle Heart Watch. Circulation *63:* 537–545 (1981).
6 Sohn, Y. H.; Boudoulas, H.; O'Neill, W.; Weissler, A. M.: Identification of patients in whom coronary bypass surgery improves survival. Circulation *64:* IV–291 (1981).
7 Pugh, B.; Platt, M. R.; Mills, L J.; et al.: Unstable angina pectoris: a randomized study of patients treated medically and surgically. Am. J. Cardiol. *41:* 1291–1298 (1978).
8 Selden, R.; Neill, W. A.; Ritzman, L.; et al.: Medical versus surgical therapy for acute coronary insufficiency. New Engl. J. Med. *293:* 1329–1334 (1975).
9 Bertolasi, C. A.; Tronge, J. E.; Carreno, C. A.; et al.: Unstable angina – prospective and randomized study of its evolution, with and without surgery. Am. J. Cardiol. *33:* 201–208 (1974).

Prof. D. H. Spodick, MD, St. Vincent Hospital, Cardiology Division,
Worcester, MA 01604 (USA)

Adv. Cardiol., vol. 31, pp. 51–59 (Karger, Basel 1982)

Coronary Bypass Surgery in Prevention of Premature Mortality

E. Varnauskas

Department of Cardiology, Sahlgrenska Hospital, Göteborg, Sweden

The question whether or not coronary bypass surgery prolongs life beyond that expected with medical management has important theoretical and practical implications.

It is well established that incapacitating angina pectoris is dramatically cured by coronary bypass surgery in most patients. It certainly works, but why? The following hypothetical mechanisms for pain relief by operation are usually suggested: (i) improved myocardial perfusion provided by a new channel bypassing the obstruction in a diseased coronary artery; (ii) denervation of the portion of the heart where pain originates; (iii) the placebo effect; (iv) infarction of the ischemic myocardium, and (v) a combination of the four above-mentioned mechanisms.

Extensive laboratory investigations of myocardial perfusion and left ventricular function before and after surgery have not as yet provided indisputable evidence to show which one of the above mechanisms is the most probable. The therapeutic implications of various mechanisms for pain relief are not equal and therefore cannot be neglected. For instance, silencing of ischemic pain may not be a worthwhile objective. Pain is a basic protective mechanism and its abolition may well prevent the patient from discountinuing the activity responsible for the ischemia [1].

If, however, aortocoronary bypass grafting is shown to prolong life, improved perfusion of the ischemic myocardium would be the most likely explanation of the analgesic effect of operation. In addition coronary bypass surgery could be then considered not only for pain relief but also for prevention of premature mortality.

The objective of this presentation is to review the evidence that coronary bypass surgery prolongs life, and to focus the attention on the types of patients who may benefit most, or least.

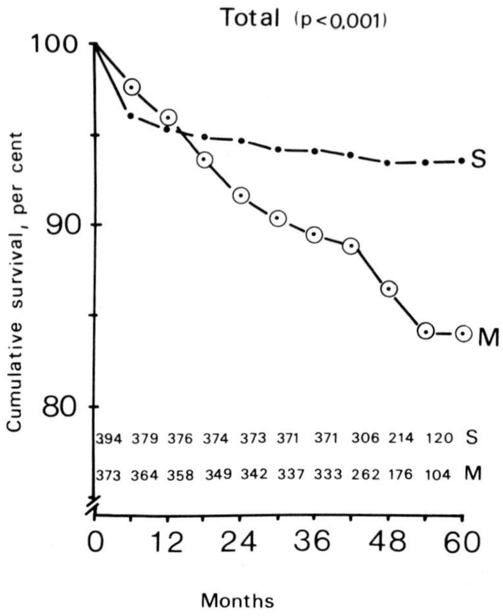

Fig. 1. The European Coronary Surgery Study [6]. Cumulative survival curves for the medical (M) and surgical (S) treatment groups of total patient population.

There are two large prospective randomized studies which have reported convincing evidence regarding coronary bypass surgery effect on survival in patients with stable angina pectoris: the Veterans Administration Study [2, 3] and the European Coronary Surgery Study [4–6]. Although the design of the two studies is similar, the criteria for patient selection are different. Further, the patients were recruited and operated between 1970 and 1974 in the VA study and between 1973 and 1976 in the European study. It is important to keep these differences in mind when comparing the results between the two studies.

A third large randomized trial – NHLBI Coronary Artery Surgery Study (CASS) – is in progress since 1975 (recruitment completed 1979); the results have not as yet been published.

I have chosen to illustrate my presentation mainly by the interim results of the European study analyzed at the minimum follow-up of 3 years [6]. When appropriate, I will compare these results with those of the VA study [2, 3].

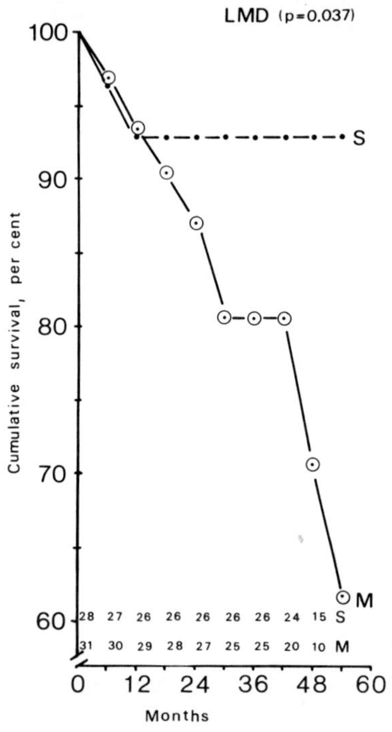

Fig. 2. The European Coronary Surgery Study [6]. Cumulative survival curves for the medical (M) and surgical (S) treatment groups of the subset of patients with left main disease (LMD).

The European study includes male patients younger than 65 years of age with stable angina pectoris of more than 3 months duration, 50% or more obstruction in at least two major coronary arteries and 50% or greater left ventricular ejection fraction. 394 of these patients were randomized into the surgical treatment group and 373 patients in the medical treatment group. The cumulative survival for these two groups extending to a 5-year follow-up is shown in figure 1. The difference between the two curves tested by log-rank test is highly significant, p value <0.001. The policy of surgical treatment is convincingly superior to that of the medical treatment.

The greatest benefit of surgical treatment policy was obtained in the subset of patients with left main disease (fig. 2) and in the subset of patients with three vessel disease (fig. 3). The p value for the difference between the two treatments was 0.037 in the left main disease subset and <0.001 in the three vessel disease subset. Although the level of significance is relatively

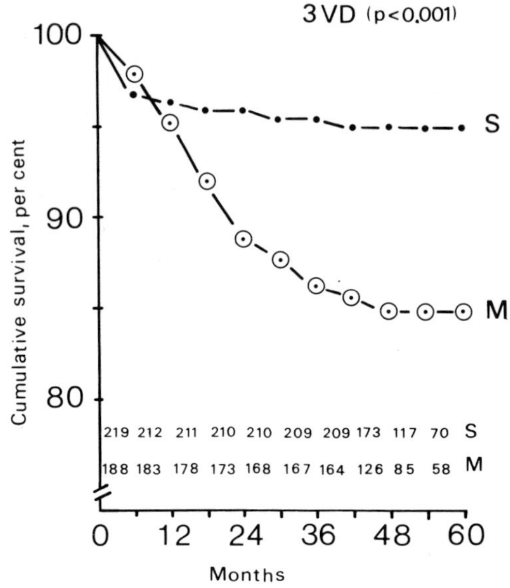

Fig. 3. The European Coronary Surgery Study [6]. Cumulative survival curves for the medical (M) and surgical (S) treatment groups of the subset of patients with three vessel disease (3VD).

low for the survival difference in the left main disease subset, the markedly higher survival for surgical patients is convincing because the difference is in the same direction as for the total patient population and the subset of patients with three vessel disease. Furthermore, this finding in patients with left main disease is in agreement with the results of the VA study [2]. Both studies included relatively small numbers of patients which also explains the relatively low level of significance for the difference between the two treatments.

Contrary to the European study the VA study failed to show significantly improved survival in surgically treated patients with three vessel disease [3]. Although the differences in patient composition between the two studies does not permit a direct comparison the cumulative survival curves for the medical patients with three vessel disease were remarkably similar in both studies. In the VA study a relatively high operative mortality does not alone explain the lack of significant difference in late survival between the two treatment groups [3].

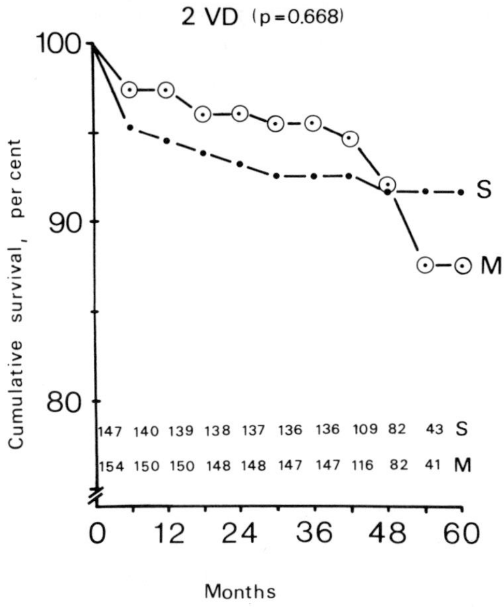

Fig. 4. The European Coronary Surgery Study [6]. Cumulative survival curves for the medical (M) and surgical (S) treatment groups of the subset of patients with two vessel disease (2VD).

Figure 4 illustrates that there is no significant difference in survival between the medical and surgical groups with two vessel disease, mainly due to excellent survival for the medically treated patients. A similar result was found in the VA study.

Further subdivision of patients with two vessel disease into two subsets by the absence or presence of narrowing in the proximal segment of left anterior descending artery (LAD) discloses that two vessel disease actually defines a prognostically heterogeneous group of patients. Comparison of the two survival curves for medically treated patients reveals that the survival is significantly superior in the subset of patients without coexistent proximal LAD lesion. On the other hand the survival difference between the two treatments is insignificant in the subsets with and without coexistent proximal LAD narrowing, respectively (fig. 5).

Figure 6 is designed to illustrate the 5-year survival rate in medically and surgically treated series of patients published between 1975 and 1981 [6–23]. Figure 6 shows that the results of the European study are in the upper range of survival both in the medical and surgical series. It also

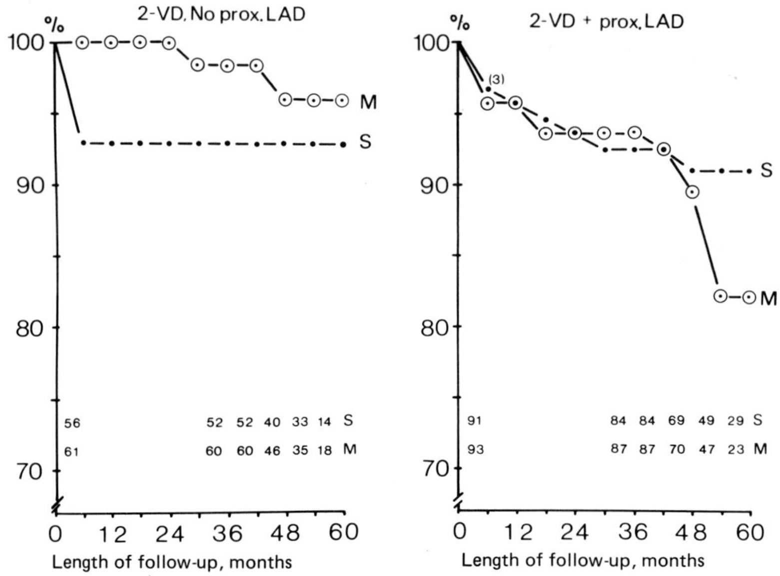

a *b*

Fig. 5. The European Coronary Surgery Study [6]. *a* Cumulative survival curves for the medical (M) and surgical (S) treatment groups of the subset of patients with 2VD and no coexistent narrowing in the proximal segment of left anterior descending artery (LAD). *b* 2VD patients with coexistent proximal LAD narrowing.

confirms that the greatest survival benefit of surgical treatment is to be expected in high risk patients, i.e. those with left main disease and three vessel disease. In low risk patients the prognosis with medical treatment is so good that it appears to be very difficult to prove that also these patients may benefit from surgery.

Exercise ECG test is one of the best noninvasive methods to identify high risk patients. Ischemic ST segment shift by 1.5 mm or more during or after exercise is known to predict poor prognosis in patients with coronary artery disease. This was also true in the European study. Coronary bypass surgery significantly improved survival in this type of patient, while it had no definite effect in patients with less pronounced ST segment shift during exercise [24].

Summarizing the so far published results of coronary bypass surgery on survival in patients with stable angina pectoris it can be concluded that: (i) coronary bypass surgery significantly improves survival in selected groups of patients; (ii) the greatest effect is achieved in high risk patients, i.e. those

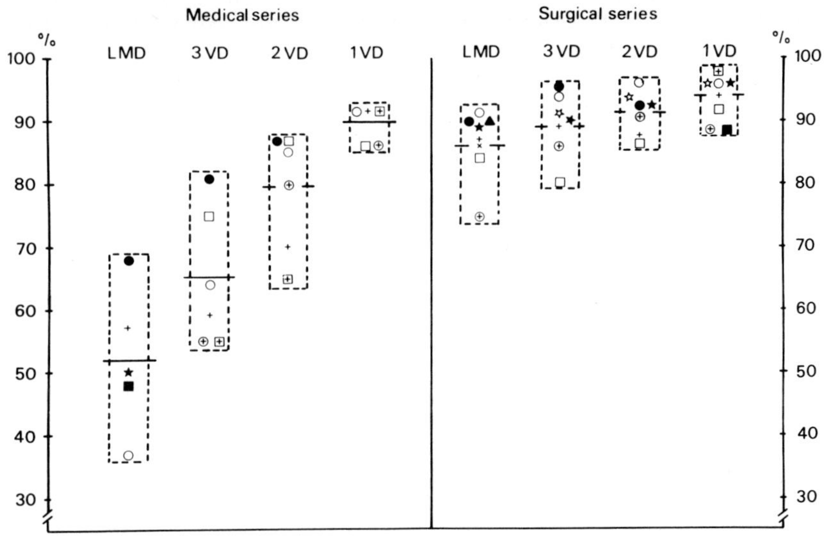

Fig. 6. Survival rate at 5-year follow-up in medical and surgical series published 1975–1981 [6–23].

with left main disease and three vessel disease; (iii) marked ischemic ST segment response (≥1.5 mm) to exercise strongly suggests that the feasibility of coronary bypass surgery should be seriously considered; (iv) there is no evidence to indicate that coronary bypass surgery improves survival in patients with single vessel disease, two vessel disease without proximal LAD narrowing and in patients with no ischemic symptoms, and (v) poor left ventricular function has an adverse influence on short- and long-term survival after surgery.

References

1 Bulkley, B. H.; Ross, R.S.: Coronary-artery bypass surgery: it works, but why? (Editorial). Ann. intern. Med. *88:* 835 (1978).

2 Takaro, T.; Hultgren, H. N.; Lipton, M. J.; Detre, K. M.: The VA cooperative randomised study of surgery for coronary arterial occlusive disease. II. Subgroup with significant left main lesions. Circulation *54:* suppl. III, pp. 107–117 (1976).

3 Murphy, M. L.; Hultgren, H. N.; Detre, K.; Thomsen, J.; Takaro, T.: Treatment of chronic stable angina: a preliminary report of survival data of the randomised Veterans Administration cooperative study. New Engl. J. Med. *297:* 621–627 (1977).

4 Varnauskas, E.; Olsson, B.: The European multicenter CABG trial; in Yu, Goodwin, Progress in cardiology, pp. 83–89, Saunders, Philadelphia (1977).
5 European Coronary Surgery Study Group: Coronary-artery bypass surgery in stable angina pectoris: survival at two years. Lancet *i:* 889–893 (1979).
6 Second Interim Report by the European Coronary Surgery Study Group: Prospective randomised study of coronary artery bypass surgery in stable angina pectoris. Lancet *ii:* 491–496 (1980).
7 Bruschke, A. V. G.: Ten-year follow-up of 601 nonsurgical cases of angiographically documented coronary disease. Angiographic correlations. Cleveland Clin. *45:* 143–144 (1978).
8 Burggraf, G. W.; Parker, J. O.: Prognosis in coronary artery disease. Angiographic, hemodynamic, and clinical factors. Circulation *51:* 146–156 (1975).
9 Campeau, L.; Corbara, F.; Crochet, D.; Petitclerc, R.: Left main coronary artery stenosis. The influence of aortocoronary bypass surgery on survival. Circulation *57:* 1111–1115 (1978).
10 Harris, P, J.; Phil, D,; Harrell, F. E.; Lee, K. L.; Behar, V. S.; Rosati, R. A.: Survival in medically treated coronary artery disease. Circulation *60:* 1259–1269 (1979).
11 Lichtlen, P. R.: Natural history of coronary artery disease based on coronary angiography. A critical review. Cleveland Clin. *45:* 153–155 (1978).
12 Lim, J. S.; Proudfit, W. L.; Sones, F. M., Jr.: Left main coronary arterial obstruction: Long-term follow-up of 141 non surgical cases. Am. J. Cardiol. *36:* 131 (1975).
13 Loop, F. D.; Sheldon, W. C.; Lytle, B. W.; Cosgrove, D. M.; Proudfit, W. L.: The efficacy of coronary artery surgery. Am. Heart J. *101:* 86–96 (1981).
14 Alderman, E. L.; Brown, C. R.; Sanders, G. R.; Stinson, E. B.: Survival following bypass graft surgery. Cleveland Clin. Q. *45:* 157–159 (1978).
15 Cameron, A.; Kemp, H. G.; Shimomura, S.; Santilli, E.; Green, G. E.; Hutchinson, J. E.; Mekhjian, H. A.: Aortoconary bypass surgery. A 7-year follow-up. Circulation *59/60:* suppl. I, pp. 9–13 (1979).
16 Farinha, J. B.; Kaplan, M. A.; Harris, C. N.; Dunne, E. F.; Carlish, R. A.; Kay, J. H.; Brooks, S.: Disease of the left main coronary artery. Surgical treatment and long-term follow up in 267 patients. Am. J. Cardiol. *42:* 124–128 (1978).
17 Greene, D. G.; Bunnell, I. L.; Arani, D. T.; Schimert, G.; Lajos, T. Z.; Lee, A. B.; Tandon, R. N.; Zimdahl, W. T.; Bozer, J. M.; Kohn, R. M.; Visco, J. P.; Dean, D. C.; Smith, G. L.: Long-term survival after coronary bypass surgery. Comparison of various subsets of patients with general population. Br. Heart J. *45:* 417–426 (1981).
18 Hoffman, R. G.; Blumlein, S. L.; Anderson, A. J.; Barboriak, J. J.; Walker, J. A.; Rimm, A. A.: The probability of surviving coronary bypass surgery. Five-year results from 1,718 patients. J. Am. med. Ass. *243:* 1341–1344 (1980).
19 Kirklin, J. W.; Kouchoukos, N. T.; Blackstone, E. H.; Oberman, A.: Research related to surgical treatment of coronary artery disease. Circulation *60:* 1613–1618 (1979).
20 Loop, F. D.; Cosgrove, D. M.; Lytle, B. W.; Thurer, R. L.; Simpfendorfer, C.; Taylor, P. C.; Proudfit, W. L.: An 11-year evolution of coronary arterial surgery (1967–1978). Ann. Surg. *190:* 444–455 (1979).
21 Loop, F. D.; Lytle, B. W.; Cosgrove, D. M.; Sheldon, W. C.; Irarrazaval, M.; Taylor, P. C.; Groves, L. K.; Pichard, A. D.: Atherosclerosis of the left main coronary artery: 5-year results of surgical treatment. Am. J. Cardiol. *44:* 195–201 (1979).

22 Tyras, D. H.; Barner, H. B.; Kaiser, G. C.; Codd, J. E.; Laks, H.; Pennington, D. G.; Willman, L.: Long-term results of myocardial revascularization. Am. J. Cardiol. *44:* 1290–1296 (1979).
23 Walker, J. A.: Survival following myocardial revascularization. An analysis at 8 years. Cleveland Clin. Q. *45:*169–171 (1977).
24 European Coronary Surgery Study Group: To be published (1982).

Prof. E. Varnauskas, MD, Department of Cardiology, Sahlgrenska Hospital, S–413 45 Göteborg (Sweden)

Adv. Cardiol., vol. 31, pp. 60–72 (Karger, Basel 1982)

Coronary Surgery as Secondary Prevention

Objectives and Achievements of Surgical Myocardial Revascularization

Joseph B. Borman[a], *Dov V. Shimon*[a], *Azai Appelbaum*[a], *Mervyn S. Gotsman*[b]

[a] Department of Cardiothoracic Surgery and [b] Cardiology Service, Hadassah University Hospital, Jerusalem, Israel

Coronary artery disease is the major cause of death in adults in Israel, with a mortality rate of more than 7,000 persons per year in a population of approximately 3.5 million.

For the last decade, we have been involved in the surgical management of patients with coronary artery disease and our cumulative experience with direct myocardial revascularization has led us to define the objectives and achievements of the surgeon in the rehabilitation of patients with ischemic heart disease.

Role of the Surgeon

(1) Relief of pain. (2) Prolongation of life. (3) Prevention of myocardial infarction. (4) Improvement of left ventricular function. (5) Suppression of ventricular arrhythmias.

Each of the above objectives will be analysed in order to assess the achievements of coronary artery bypass surgery (CABS).

Relief of Pain

There is general agreement that anginal pain is substantially relieved in the majority of patients undergoing operation: at 5 years following CABS, 60% of the patients are completely relieved of pain, and about 90% are

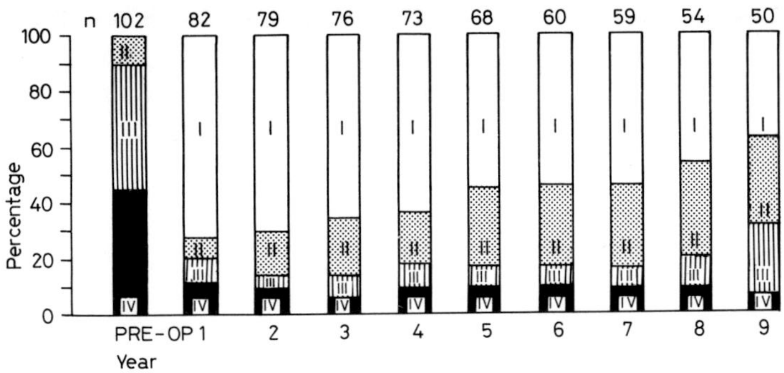

Fig. 1. New York Heart Association functional class in the preoperative period (PRE-OP) and in the subsequent postoperative years. The number of patients in each year is indicated. Preoperatively, all patients were symptomatic and 89% had class III or IV angina. Postoperatively, 75% of the surviving patients were asymptomatic at 1 year, 53% at 5 years and 34% at 9 years [from ref. 7 with permission].

improved. *Mundth and Austen* [1] reported 60–70% of 10,000 patients operated before 1971, to be in class I NYHA. *Hurst* et al. [2] quoted 62% as being in class I NYHA whilst 92% were improved. The Cleveland Clinic group [3] found 65–69% to be without angina at 5 years postsurgery.

The degree of pain depends on (1) complete revascularisation; (2) patency of the grafts; (3) progression of coronary artery disease, and (4) other types of chest pain. *Sheldon* et al. [4] reported 87% of patients asymptomatic at 4 years if completely revascularised, compared to 56% in whom only partial revascularisation had been carried out.

Our own experience in Jerusalem typifies the move to more complete revascularisation (in vessels larger than 1 mm in diameter). In 1973, only 72.1% of graftable vessels were bypassed, in 1975 it amounted to 82.5%, rising to 97.6% in 1979 and stabilising at 98.6% in 1980. Recent reports from other workers confirm this trend. *Askins and Austen* [5] attained an increase from 3.3 grafts per patient in 1979 to 3.8 grafts per patient in 1980; *Loop* et al. [6] showed an increase from 1.5 grafts per patient in 1967 to 2.5 grafts per patient in 1978. On the other hand, long-term follow-up reveals a very gradual erosion of the excellent results achieved by surgery in the relief of anginal pain. *Buda* et al. [7] showed that 73% of 102 patients were in class I NYHA at one year post operatively, but there was a slow attrition thereafter, so that at nine years only 34% had remained asymptomatic (fig. 1). This finding may be explained by changes in the vein grafts due, mainly

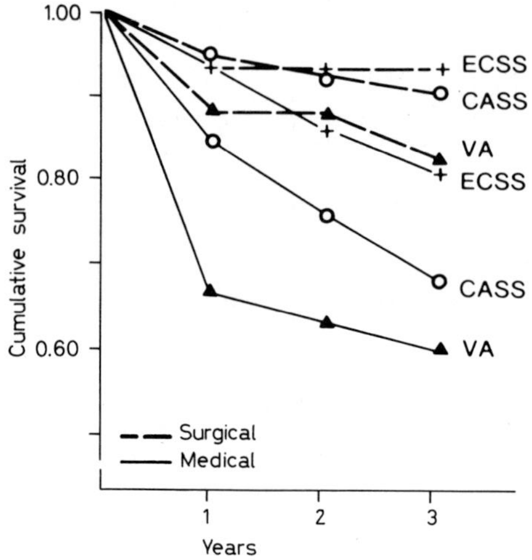

Fig. 2. Left main coronary artery disease – medical vs. surgical survival in three major prospective studies. Comparison of medical (—) vs. surgical cumulative (- - -) survival in patients with significant left main coronary artery disease in three major prospective studies, showing improved survival after 3 years in each study [from ref. 13–15].

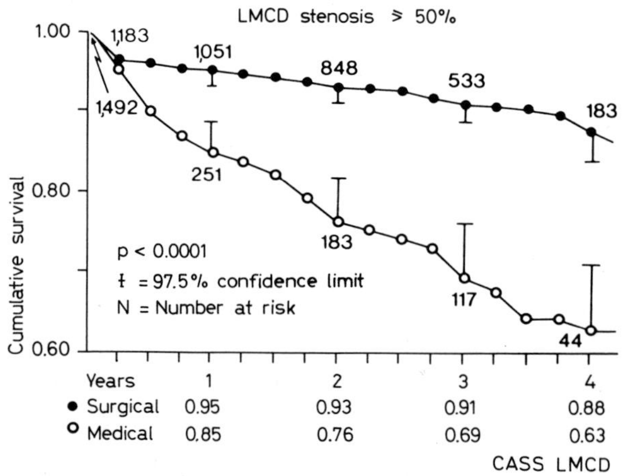

Fig. 3. Cumulative survival (actuarial method) in surgical (●) vs. medical (○) cohorts [from ref. 15 with permission].

to fibrous intimal hyperplasia. *Kouchoukos* et al. [8] report a 1.7% annual graft attrition rate, *Grondin* et al [9], mentioned 3–5%, *Lawrie* et al. [10] found 3.2% and *Hamby* et al. [11] quote 3.2% per year. *Kouchoukos* et al. [12] similarly reported a slow deterioration in vein graft patency over a 5-year period.

Prolongation of Life

Left Main Disease

Again there is little controversy regarding the value of surgery in the management of patients with significant (greater than 50%) narrowing of the left main coronary vessel. Three separate prospective studies prove the superiority of surgical therapy [13–15] (fig. 2). A breakdown of the CASS results over a 4-year period emphasises the improved survival with surgery at every time stage ($p < 0.0001$; fig. 3).

Kirklin et al. [16] have compared the cumulative survival of 247 patients operated for left main disease with a population matched for age and sex. Survival of the surgical cohort over the 5-year period of the comparison was only marginally inferior to that of the general population.

Triple Vessel Disease

Results of surgery in 216 patients operated for triple vessel disease at Buffalo General Hospital were compared with medically treated patients from five different centers [17]. Cumulative mortality in the medically treated series was uniformly higher over the 5-year period of the comparison.

Kirklin et al. [16] compared results of surgery in patients with triple vessel disease who were operated with a group of patients who were surgical candidates but who were not operated. Again, the survival figures of those operated were demonstratively higher [16] (fig. 4). The same trend became apparent in a similar study group of patients with double vessel disease (fig. 5, 6).

The Cleveland Clinic group compared 5-year survivals of medically and surgically treated patients with single, double and triple vessel disease [18]. Little difference was noted with single vessel disease, but in those with double and particularly triple vessel narrowing, survival was much increased in the surgical subset. This finding continued to be positive when follow-up was extended to 10 years (fig. 7).

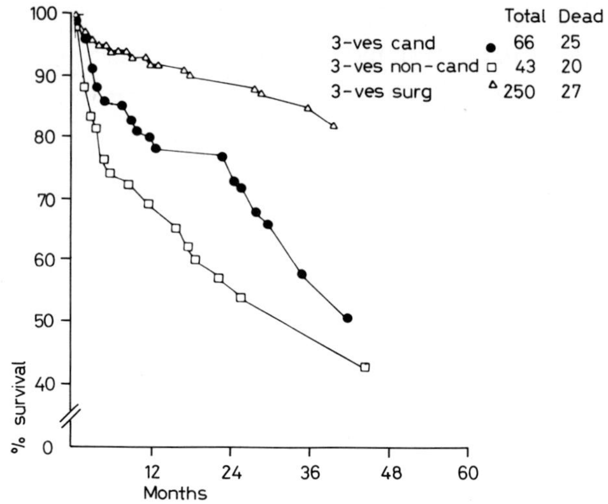

Fig. 4. Comparison between three groups of patients with 3-vessel coronary artery disease from the University of Alabama series: 250 surgical patients (△), 43 patients treated medically only because of unsuitable coronary anatomy (□), and 66 patients with surgically compatible anatomy who were not operated (●). Markedly improved survival is noted in the surgical group [from ref. 16 with permission].

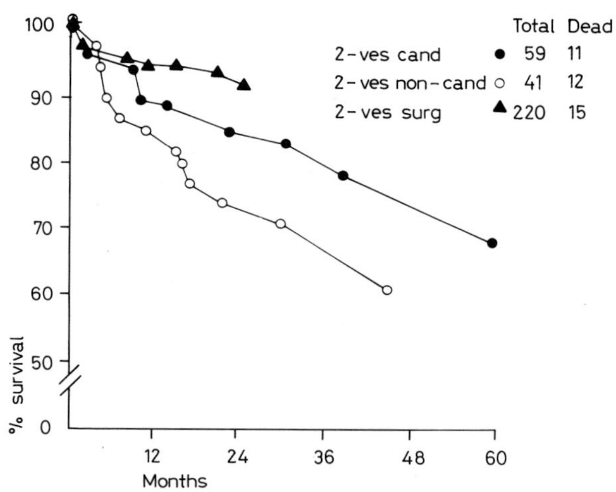

Fig. 5. As in figure 4 for patients with two vessel disease [from ref. 16 with permission].

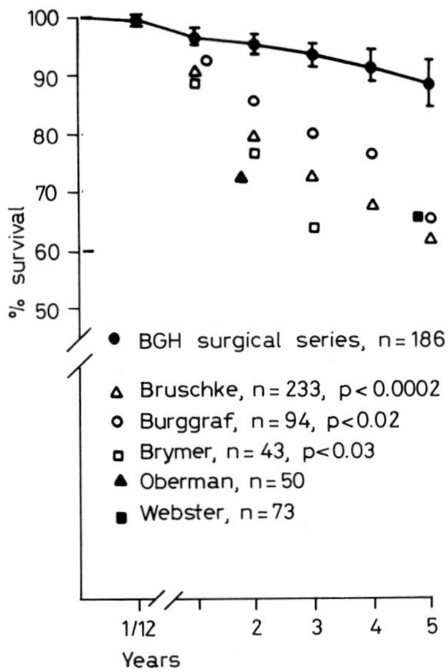

Fig. 6. Comparison between 186 surgical patients with double vessel coronary artery disease from the Buffalo General Hospital and five groups of similar patients treated medically only [from ref. 17 with permission].

There appears to be strong evidence at present that surgery prolongs life in patients with significant left main disease and in those with triple and severe double vessel disease. As stated by *Hurst* et al. [2]: 'None of the available studies show that modern medical treatment is superior to bypass surgery in prolonging life. A few studies show that the two methods of treatment are of equal value, but the majority show the superiority of bypass surgery to medical treatment in prolonging life'

Prevention of Myocardial Infarction

Stable Angina

Mason et al. [19] compared the incidence of myocardial infarction in patients with stable angina who had undergone surgery and medically treated cases. Over a follow-up period averaging 2.6 years, both total and fatal infarction rate was significantly lower in patients who had had coronary artery bypass (fig. 8).

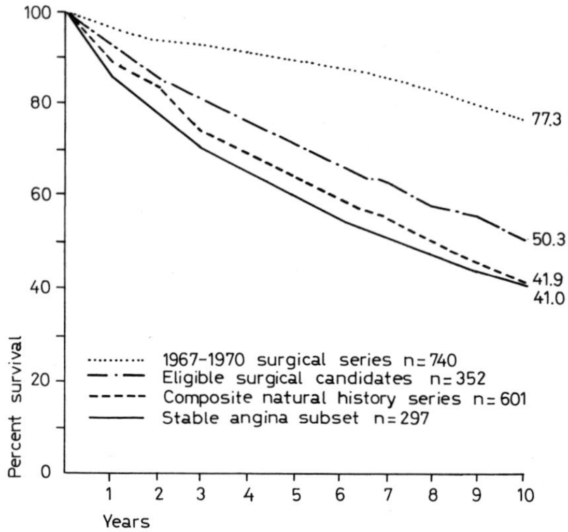

Fig. 7. 10-year survival of 740 patients who underwent coronary bypass grafting only, from May 1967 until December 1970, in the Cleveland Clinic. The 10-year survival of 77 % is compared with (1) 601 patients in composite natural history studies published by *Proudfit* et al. [progr. cardiovasc. Dis. *21:* 53, 1978]; (2) a subset of 352 eligible surgical candidates (left main stenosis of more than 50 % excluded); (3) a subset of patients with chronic stable angina [from ref. 3 with permission].

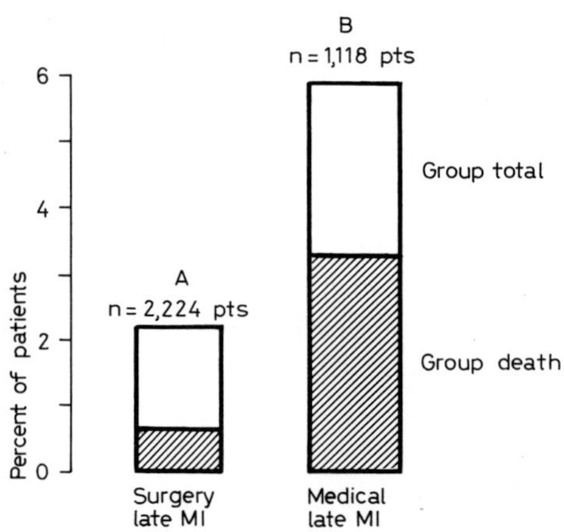

Fig. 8. The annual incidences of total and fatal myocardial infarction (MI) in surgically treated stable angina patients (derived from eight surgical reports that average a follow-up of 2.6 years) are compared to the same end points from three natural history studies. Late infarction in the surgical patients was 2.1 % per year, with a 0.6 % annual rate of fatal late infarction. Medically treated stable anginal patients show incidences of 5.9 % annual MI and 3.5 % fatal infarction [modified from ref. 19].

Table I. Coronary artery bypass surgery: hospital mortality and myocardial infarction rates for medically treated patients with unstable angina

Report	Number of patients	Deaths n	Deaths %	Myocardial infarctions n	Myocardial infarctions %
Bender et al. [25]	35	2	6	5	14
Berk et al. [26]	21	4	19	13	62
Bertolasi et al. [27]	51	6	12	10	20
Fischl et al. [28]	23	1	4	4	17
Fulton et al. [29]	167	3	2	23	14
Hultgren et al. [30]	66	14	21	11	17
Krauss et al. [31]	100	3	3	7	7
Matloff et al. [32]	35	14	40	31	90
NCSG [33]	147	4	3	12	8
Neil et al. [34]	20	0	0	2	10
Scanlon et al. [35]	31	6	19	22	71
Total	696	57	8.2 (range 0–40%)	140	20.1 (range 7–90%)

NCSG = National cooperative study group.

Unstable Angina

A random selection of recent reports concerning the medical treatment of unstable angina including 696 patients, revealed an average infarction rate of 20.1%. Mortality in this subset was 8.2% (table I).

Opposed to this, random selection of 14 reports of surgical therapy inclusive of 1,454 patients demonstrated an incidence of myocardial infarction of 11.9% and a mortality figure of 4.8% (table II).

There appears to be little doubt that in both stable and unstable angina, surgery is more effective in preventing myocardial infarction. Furthermore, fatality figures are lower in those operated as compared to the nonsurgically managed patients.

Improvement in Left Ventricular Function

Ahmed et al. [20] studied 39 patients with unstable angina and found that left ventricular ejection fraction at rest improved after surgery from an average of 0.59 to 0.69. *Freeman* et al. [21] were unable to demonstrate

Table II. Coronary artery bypass surgery: hospital mortality and myocardial infarction rates for surgically treated patients with unstable angina

Report	Number of patients	Deaths n	Deaths %	Myocardial infarctions n	Myocardial infarctions %
Ahmed et al. [36]	71	3	4	5	7
Bender et al. [25]	53	3	6	6	11
Bertolasi et al. [27]	62	4	6	8	13
Cohn et al. [37]	127	5	4	10	8
Golding et al. [38]	100	4	4	18	18
Hultgren et al. [30]	52	3	6	10	19
Langon et al. [39]	123	5	4	22	18
Levine et al. [40]	60	2	3	1	2
Matloff et al. [32]	88	3	3	8	9
NCSG [33]	141	7	5	24	17
Olinger et al. [41]	95	1	1	3	3
Schroeder et al. [42]	80	7	9	13	16
Seybold-Epting et al. [43]	302	20	7	33	11
Wysham and Rogers [44]	100	0	0	13	13
Total	1,454	67	4.6 (range 0–9%)	174	11.9 (range 2–19%)

NCSG = National cooperative study group.

improvement in left ventricular ejection fraction at rest after surgery. On the other hand, ejection fraction was shown to increase during exercise in patients after coronary artery bypass (fig. 9).

A computerised 3-dimensional tracing of left ventricular contraction in a patient before and after triple bypass for unstable angina is shown in figure 10. It is quite obvious that both global and regional contraction has increased markedly following operation. Another patient with very poor left ventricular function (EF 0.20) was studied by radionucleide scanning (MUGA) before and after surgery with atrial pacing at identical rates. Both the RAO and LAO views demonstrate improved left ventricular function after surgery. Whereas EF dropped to 0.11 before surgery, it increased to 0.29 after bypass. Thallium scan in the same patient clearly shows improved perfusion of the septal and apical regions of the left ventricle after operation.

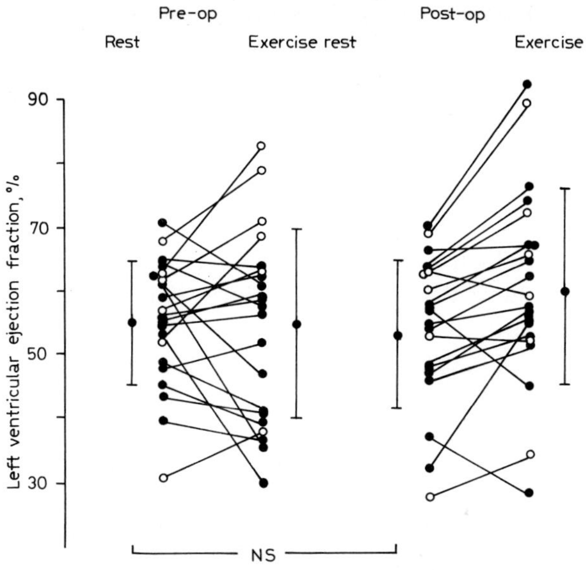

Fig. 9. The exercise response of left ventricular ejection fraction in each patient before and after surgery. Mean values and standard deviation are shown. ○ = Patients with normal response before surgery; ● = patients with abnormal response before surgery [from ref. 21 with permission].

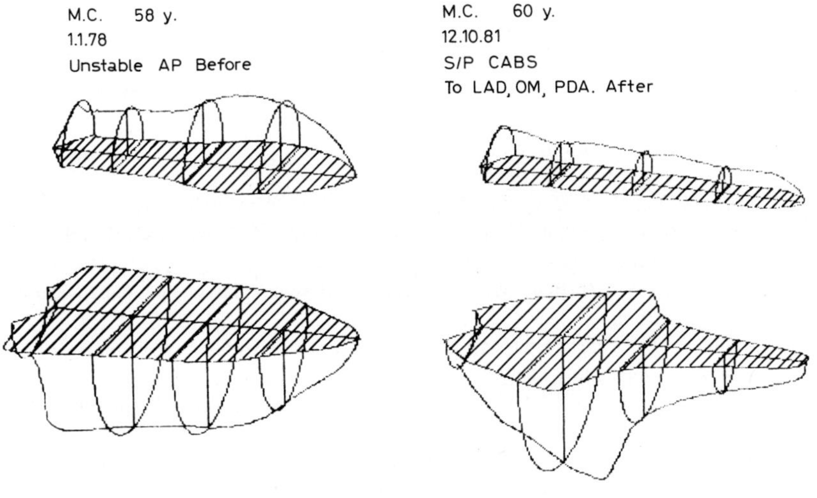

Fig. 10. Preoperative and postoperative computerized three-dimensional tracing of RAO view of left ventricular angiography. The left ventricle is divided into eight segments. Improved contraction is noted in most segments, mainly apical and infero-apical.

Suppression of Arrhythmias (Surgical Possibilities)

(1) Myocardial revascularisation. (2) Left ventricular aneurysmectomy (or scar resection). (3) Encircling endocardial ventriculotomy (EEV) or endocardial resection.

The role of myocardial revascularisation without additional resectional procedures in the control of ventricular arrhythmias is uncertain at present. A prospective study of sudden death occurrence in patients with multiple coronary artery disease shows that following surgery, 7 of 121 patients died suddenly. 23 of 96 patients treated conservatively for a similar period averaging 39 months died suddenly [22]. Assuming that ventricular arrhythmia was the cause of death in some instances, the figures impressively favour surgery. *Hart* et al. [23] recently reported 42 patients treated with coronary artery bypass for problematic ventricular arrhythmias. During a 5-year follow-up, survival was 86% and only one death could be attributed to arrhythmias. Contrarily, *Buda* et al. [24] do not recommend bypass grafting without myocardial resection for refractory ventricular arrhythmias.

References

1 Mundth, E. D.; Austen,W. G.: Surgical measures for coronary artery disease. New Engl. J. Med. *293:* 124 (1975).

2 Hurst, J. W.; King, S. B.; Logue, R. B.; et al.: Value of coronary bypass surgery: Controversies in cardiology. Part I. A. J. Cardiol. *42:* 308 (1978).

3 Loop, F. D.; Sheldon, W. C.; Lytle, B. W.; et al.: The efficacy of coronary artery surgery. Am. Heart J. *101:* 86 (1981).

4 Sheldon, W. C.; Rincon, G.; Pichard, A. D.; et al.: Surgical treatment of coronary artery disease. Pure graft operations with a study of 741 patients followed 3–7 years. Progr. cardiovasc. Dis. *18:* 237 (1975).

5 Akins, A. W.; Austen, W. G.: Myocardial revascularization. Curr. Probl. Surg. (January 1981).

6 Loop, F. D.; Cosgrove, D. M.; Lytle, B. W.; et al.: An 11-year evaluation of coronary arterial surgery (1967–1978). Ann. Surg. *190:* 444 (1979).

7 Buda, A. J.; Macdonald I. L.; Anderson, M. J.; et al.: Long-term results following coronary bypass operation. J. thorac. cardiovasc. Surg. *82:* 383 (1981).

8 Kouchoukos, N. T.; Karp, R. B.; Oberman, A.; et al.: Long-term patency of saphenous veinsfor coronary bypass grafting. Circulation *58:* suppl. 1, p. 96 (1978).

9 Grondin, C. M.; Lesperance, J.; Bourassa, M. G.; et al.: Coronary artery grafting with the saphenous vein or internal mammary artery. Comparison of late results in two consecutive series of patients. Ann. thorac. Surg. *20:* 605 (1975).

10 Lawrie, G. M.; Lie, J.; Morris, G. C.; et al.: Vein graft patency and intimal proliferation after aortocoronary bypass: Early and long-term angiopathologic correlations. Am. J. Cardiol. *38:* 856 (1976).

11 Hamby, R. I.; Aintalbian, A.; Handler, M.; et al.: Aortocoronary saphenous vein bypass grafts. Long-term patency, morphology and blood flow in patients with patent grafts after surgery. Circulation *60:* 901 (1979).

12 Kouchoukos, N. T.; Kirklin, J.W.; Oberman, A.: An appraisal of coronary bypass grafting. Circulation *50:* 11 (1974).

13 ECSS-European Coronary Surgery Study Group: Coronary-artery bypass surgery in stable angina pectoris. Survival at two years. Lancet *1:* 889 (1979).

14 Kennedy, J.W.; Kaiser, G. C.; Fisher, L. D.; et al.: Multivariate discriminant analysis of the clinical and angiographic prediction of operative mortality from the Collaborative Study in Coronary Artery Surgery (CASS). J. thorac, cardiovasc. Surg. *80:* 876 (1980).

15 Murphy, M. L.; Hultgren, H. N.; Detre, K.; et al.: Treatment of chronic stable angina (VA study). New Engl. J. Med. *297:* 621 (1977).

16 Kirklin, J. W.; Kouchoukos, N. T.; Blackstone, E. H.; et al.: Research related to surgical treatment of coronary artery disease. Circulation *60:* 1613 (1979).

17 Greene, D. G.; Bunnel, I. L.; Arani, D. T.: Long-term survival after coronary bypass surgery. Buffalo General Hospital, State University of New York. Brochure for Exhibit at the American Heart Ass. Meet. 1977.

18 Loop, F. D.; Sheldon, W. C.; Lytle, B. W.; et al.: The efficacy of coronary artery surgery. Am. Heart J. *101:* 86 (1981).

19 Mason, D. T.; Amsterdam, E. A.; De-Maria, A. N.; et al.: The prevention of myocardial infarction by coronary bypass surgery; in Hurst, The heart. Update II. p. 108 (McGraw-Hill, New York 1980).

20 Ahmed, M.; Thompson, R.; Seabra-Gomez, R.; et al.: Unstable angina: A clinicoarteriographic and long-term results of early myocardial revascularization. J. thorac. cardiovasc. Surg. *79:* 609 (1980).

21 Freeman, M. R.; Gray, R. J.; Berman, D. S.; et al.: Improvement in global and segmental left ventricular function after coronary bypass surgery. Circulation *64:* suppl. 2, p. 34 (1981).

22 Vismara, L. A.; Miller, R. R.; Price, J. E.; et al.: Improved longevity due to reduction of sudden death by aortocoronary bypass in coronary atherosclerosis. Am. J. Cardiol. *39:* 919 (1977).

23 Hart, N. J.; Hobbs, R. E.; Young, S. P.; et al.: Coronary artery bypass surgery and ventricular arrhythmias; in Hurst, The heart. Update IV (McGraw-Hill, New York 1981).

24 Buda, A. J.; Stinson, E. B.; Harrison, D. C.: Surgery for life-threatening ventricular tachyarrhythmias. Am. J. Cardiol. *44:* 1171 (1979).

25 Bender, H. W.; Fisher, R. D.; Faulkner, S. L.; et al.: Unstable coronary artery disease. Comparison of medical and surgical management. Ann. thorac. Surg. *19:* 521 (1975).

26 Berk, G.; Koplitt, M.; Padmanabhan, V.; et al.: Management of preinfarction angina. Evaluation and comparison of medical versus surgical therapy in 43 patients. J. thorac. cardiovasc. Surg. *71:* 110 (1976).

27 Bertolasi, C. A.; Tronge, J. E.; Riccitelli, M. A.; et al.: Natural history of unstable angina with medical or surgical therapy. Chest *70:* 596 (1976).

28 Fischl, S. J.; Herman, M. V.; Gorlin, R.: The intermediate coronary syndrome. Clinical, angiographic and therapeutic aspects. New Engl. J. Med. *288:* 1193 (1973).
29 Fulton, M,; Lutz, W.; Donald, K. W.: Natural history of unstable angina. Lancet *i:* 860 (1972).
30 Hultgren, H. N.; Pfeifer, J. R.; Angel, W. W.; et al.: Unstable angina. Comparison of medical and surgical management. Am. J. Cardiol. *39:* 734 (1977).
31 Krauss, K. R.; Hutter, A. M.; DeSanctis, R. W.: Acute coronary insufficiency: Course of follow-up. Circulation *45:* suppl. 1, p. 66 (1972).
32 Matloff, J. M.; Sustaita, H.; Chatterjee, K.; et al.: The rationale for surgery in preinfarction angina. J. thorac. cardiovasc. Surg. *69:* 73 (1976).
33 National Cooperative Study Group: Unstable angina pectoris. National Cooperative Study Group to compare surgical and medical therapy. Am. J. Cardiol. *42:* 839 (1978).
34 Neil, W. A.; Ritzmann, L. W.; Okies, J. E.; et al.: Medical vs. urgent surgical therapy for acute coronary insufficiency. A randomized study. Cardiovasc. Clin. *8:* 179 (1977).
35 Scanlon, P. J.; Nemickas, R.; Moran, J. F.; et al.: Accelerated angina pectoris. Clinical, hemodynamic, arteriographic and therapeutic experience in 85 patients. Circulation *47:* 19 (1973).
36 Ahmed, M.; Thompson, R.; Seabra-Gomes, R.; et al.: Unstable angina. A clinicoarteriographic correlation and long-term results of early myocardial revascularization. J. thorac, cardiovasc. Surg. *79:* 609 (1980).
37 Cohn, L. H.; Alpert, J.; Koster, J. K.; et al.: Changing indication for the surgical treatment of unstable angina. Archs Surg. *113:* 1312 (1978).
38 Golding, L. A. R.; Loop, F. D.; Peter, M.; et al.: Late survival following use of intraaortic balloon pump in revascularization operations. Ann. thorac. Surg. *30:* 48 (1980).
39 Langon, R. A.; Wiles, J. C.; Cohen, L. S.: Coronary surgery for unstable angina pectoris. Br. Heart J. *40:* 767 (1978).
40 Levine, F. H.; Gold, H. K.; Leinbach, R. C.; et al.: Safe early revascularization for continuing ischemia after acute myocardial infarction. Circulation *60:* suppl. 1, p. 5 (1979).
41 Olinger, G. N.; Bonchek, L. I.; Keelon, M. H.; et al.: Unstable angina pectoris – the case for operation. Am. J. Cardiol. *42:* 634 (1978).
42 Schroeder, J. S.; Lamb, I.; Hu, M.; et al.: Coronary bypass surgery for unstable angina pectoris. J. Am. med Ass. *237:* 2609 (1977).
43 Seybold-Epting, W.; Oglietty, J.; Wukasch, D. C.; et al.: Early and late results after surgical treatment of preinfarction angina. Ann. thorac. Surg. *21:* 97 (1976).
44 Wysham, D. N.; Rogers, W. R.; Coronary bypass surgery for unstable angina – a five year follow-up. Archs Surg. *114:* 611 (1979).

J. B. Borman, MD, Department of Cardiothoracic Surgery,
Hadassah University Hospital, Jerusalem (Israel)

Adv. Cardiol., vol. 31, pp. 73–79 (Karger, Basel 1982)

Long-Term Effect of Aortocoronary Bypass Surgery on Exercise Tolerance and Vocational Rehabilitation

H. Gohlke, H. Roskamm, L. Samek, K. Schnellbacher, M. Schmuziger
Rehabilitationszentrum für Herz- und Kreislaufkranke
(Ärztlicher Direktor: Prof. Dr. *H. Roskamm*), Bad Krozingen, BRD

There is not much data available on how long objective improvement of exercise capacity is maintained after bypass surgery [1, 2], and there is considerable controversy whether the improved exercise capacity and return-to-work rates are related to each other [3, 7].

Our study attempts to answer the following questions: (1) For how long is the improved exercise tolerance maintained after bypass surgery? (2) How does the return-to-work rate change over time? (3) Is there a correlation between improved exercise tolerance and return-to-work?

Between 1973 and 1978, 902 patients were operated. During operation and during the 1- to 7-year follow-up, 7% of these patients died. This study deals with 467 patients who were 55 years or younger at the time of surgery. The study population of age 55 or younger at the time of surgery was chosen to exclude patients who would retire because of reaching the age limit rather than for medical reasons within the follow-up period.

All patients had undergone preoperative exercise testing and postoperative exercise testing at 1 year after surgery. In addition, 2 exercise tests per patient were performed during the 2- to 5-year follow-up period. All exercise tests were performed with a bicycle ergometer in the supine position. Exercise was begun with 25 or 50 W and the work-load was increased every 6 min by 25 or 50 W until fatigue, severe dyspnea, angina pectoris, 80% of the age-predicted maximal heart rate, or more than 0.4 mV of ST-segment depression occurred. 12.4% of the patients had one-vessel disease, 32.5% two-vessel disease, 54.9% three-vessel disease, and 13.5% of the patients had a more than 50% stenosis of the left main stem. The preoperative exercise tolerance of these patients was 62 W (fig. 1). The angina-free work-load was 41 W.

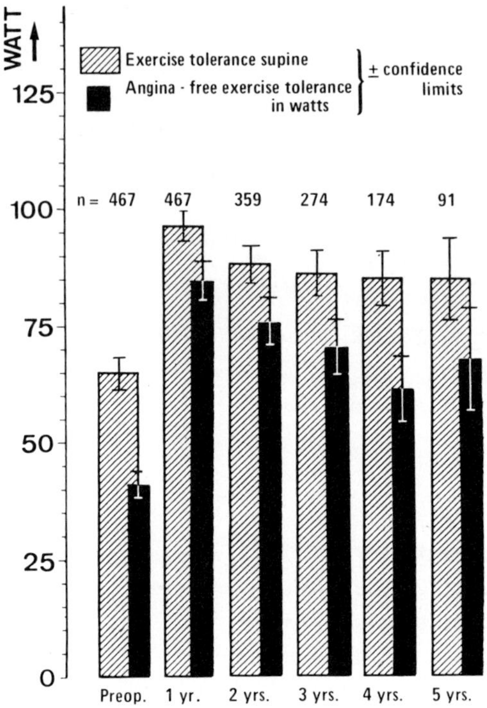

Fig. 1. Maximum exercise tolerance and angina-free exercise tolerance (in Watts) before and 1–5 years after surgery.

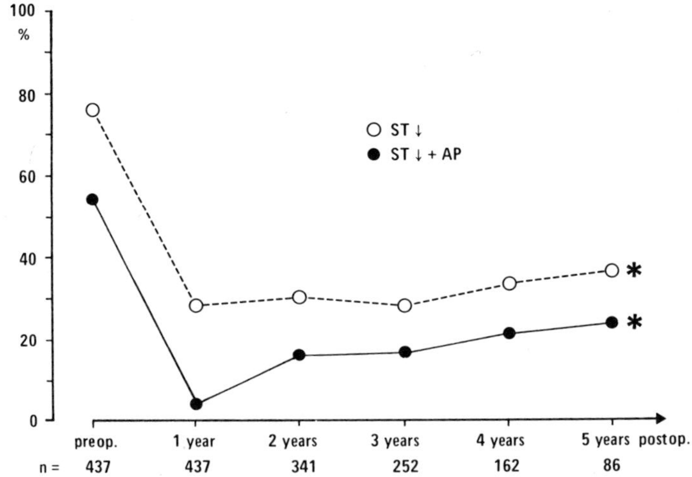

Fig. 2. Percentage of patients with ST-segment depression (open circles) and patients with ST-segment depression and angina pectoris (closed circles) before and 1–5 years after surgery; $^*p < 0.00001$ compared to preoperation.

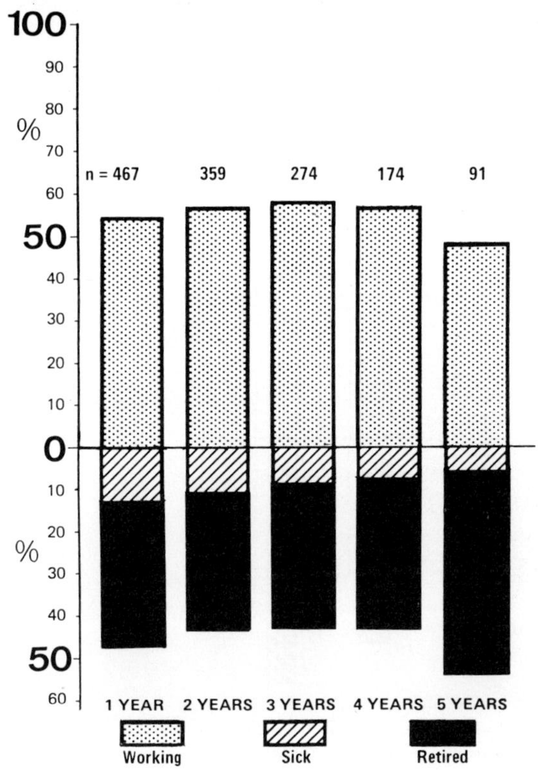

Fig. 3. Working status 1–5 years after bypass surgery.

1 year after surgery the angina-free exercise tolerance was more than doubled and the maximal exercise tolerance increased by more then 50%. Both, the maximal exercise tolerance and the angina-free exercise tolerance decreased slowly from 1 to 5 years after surgery as compared to preoperatively. The percentage of patients developing ≥ 0.1 mV ST-segment depression during exercise at 1–5 years after surgery is shown in figure 2; also shown is the percentage of patients developing moderate or severe angina pectoris in addition to ST-segment depression. Although the percentage of patients with angina pectoris and ST-segment depression increased slowly during follow-up, the occurrence of angina pectoris and ST-segment depression at 5 years after surgery is significantly lower despite

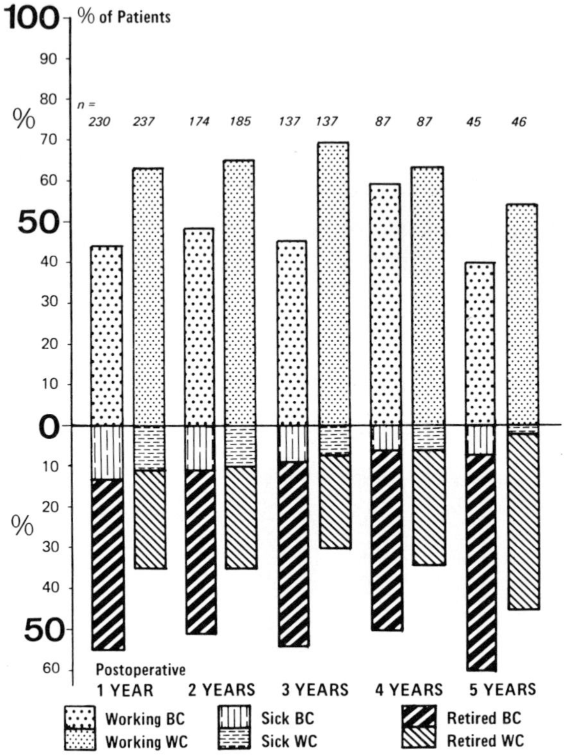

Fig. 4. Working status in blue-collar (left columns) and white-collar workers (right columns) 1–5 years after surgery.

a higher work-load. Thus, sequential exercise tests showed that there is slow and gradual loss of improvement of the exercise parameters reflecting increasing ischemia, which may be due to graft occlusion or progression of the disease in the native circulation or a combination of the two.

The work status of our 467 patients from 1 to 5 years after surgery is shown in figure 3. Approximately 50–55 % of patients are back to full-time work from 1 to 4 years after surgery, and slightly less than 50 % of patients at 5 years after surgery. The percentage of patients being retired increases slowly. The reported return-to-work rates in larger series from the United States [3, 8, 10] are significantly higher than in series reported in the German literature, and also higher than in our own experience. This is probably due to a difference in the social system; particularly the social

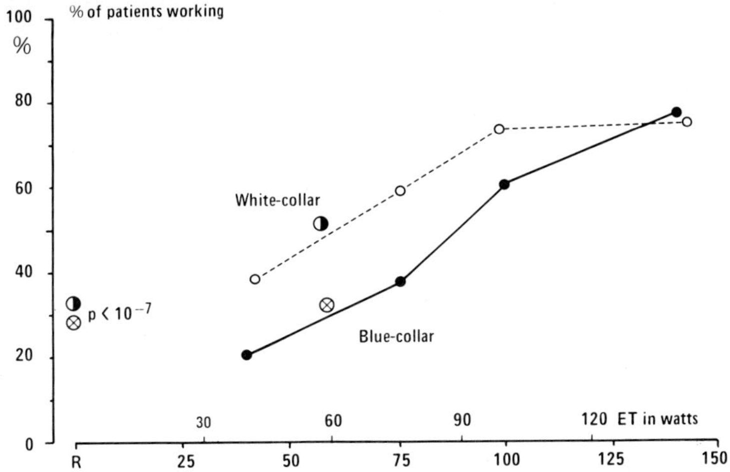

Fig. 5. Postoperative working status in relation to postoperative exercise tolerance in blue- and white-collar workers. ET = Exercise tolerance.

benefits the patient can expect after early retirement appear to play a dominant role in our experience and that of others [6].

To determine the influence of physical job demands on the return-to-work rate, the work status after surgery was determined in blue-collar and white-collar workers (fig. 4). Prior to surgery and postoperatively these two groups did not differ significantly with respect to age and medical parameters. The percentage of patients working was consistently lower in the blue-collar worker group. A correlation of the postoperative exercise tolerance with the percentage of patients back to work is shown in figure 5 for blue and white-collar workers, respectively. There is a highly significant correlation between exercise tolerance and the return-to-work rate throughout the entire follow-up period for blue-collar workers and also for white-collar workers (fig. 5). Below an exercise tolerance of 120 W after surgery, blue-collar workers have a 10–20% lower return-to-work rate than white-collar workers with a similar exercise tolerance. When the exercise tolerance exceeded 120 W, the difference in return-to-work is no longer existent: 75% of patients are back to work after surgery in both groups.

Previous publications could not show a significant influence of the medical outcome after bypass surgery on the return-to-work rate [5, 6]. Our results differ from these reports in the literature and indicate that within the

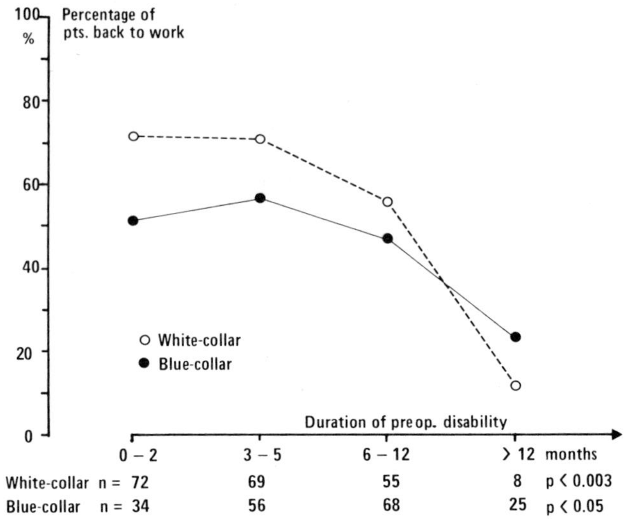

Fig. 6. The return-to-work rate in relation to the preoperative duration of disability in blue-collar and white-collar workers.

framework of a comprehensive rehabilitation program the medical outcome after aortocoronary bypass surgery had a highly significant influence on the return-to-work rate. This can be considered a success of rehabilitation that is oriented toward the functional evaluation of the patient.

In both groups, blue-collar workers and white-collar workers, there was an inverse relationship between the duration of preoperative disability and the return-to-work rate (fig. 6): the longer the disability before surgery, the less likely was a return-to-work after surgery. *David* [9] also reported that the return-to-work rate varied from 77% in patients who were less than 3 months disabled before surgery as compared to 39% in patients who were disabled for more than 6 months before surgery. *Liddle* [8] reported that only 25% of his patients were disabled for more than 2 months before surgery; in our study 83% of patients were disabled for more than 2 months before surgery, on the average for 6.5 months. A change in the decision-making process and better availability of coronary bypass surgery may be necessary to improve this. Of course there are other factors that influence return-to-work such as age, educational level, the attitude of the employer, the motivation of the individual patients, the retirement benefits, the medical insurance system and the current unemployment rate.

References

1 Frick, M. H.; Harjola, P. T.; Valle, M.: Long-term effect of coronary bypass surgery on exercise tolerance: a two-year randomized study; in Roskamm, Schmuziger, Coronary heart surgery, a rehabilitation measure, pp. 279–284 (Springer, Berlin 1979).

2 Weiner, D. A.; McCabe, C. H.; Roth, R. L.; Cutler, S. S.; Berger, R. L.; Ryan, T. J.: Serial exercise testing after coronary artery bypass surgery. Am. Heart J. *101:* 149–154 (1981).

3 Lawrie, G. M.; Morris, G. C.; Howell, J. F.; Ogura, J. W.; Spencer, W. H.; Cashion, W. R.; Winters, W. L.; Beazley, H. L.; Chapman, D. W.; Peterson, P. K.; Lie, J. T.: Results of aorto-coronary bypass more than 5 years after operation in 434 patients. Am. J. Cardiol. *40:* 665–672 (1977).

4 Wallwork, J.; Potter, B.; Caves, P. K.: Return to work after coronary artery surgery for angina. Br. med. J. *ii:* 1680–1681 (1978).

5 Lichtlen, P.; Liese, W.; Leitz, K.; Borst, H. G.: Postoperative Klinik nach aorto-koronarem Venenbypass in Relation zum Ausmass der Revaskularisation. Z. Kardiol. *67:* 83–91 (1978).

6 Blümchen, G.; Scharf-Bornhofen, E.; Brandt, D.; Van den Bergh, C.; Bierck, G.: Clinical results and social implications in patients after coronary bypass surgery; in Roskamm, Schmuziger, Coronary heart surgery, a rehabilitation measure, pp. 370–374 (Springer, Berlin 1979).

7 Oberman, A.; Kouchoukos, N. T.: Working status of patients following coronary bypass surgery. Am. Heart J. *98:* 132–133 (1979).

8 Liddle, H. V.: Perspectives in coronary artery surgery. J. thorac. cardiovasc. Surg. *81:* 1–10 (1981).

9 David, P.: Contributing factors preventing return to work of cardiac surgery patients; in Roskamm, Schmuziger, Coronary heart surgery, a rehabilitation measure, pp. 370–374 (Springer, Berlin 1979).

10 Hammermeister, K. E.; De Rouen, T. A.; English, M. T.; Dodge, H. T.: The effect of surgical versus medical therapy on return to work. Am. J. Cardiol. *44:* 105–111 (1979).

Prof. H. Roskamm, Benedikt Kreutz Rehabilitationszentrum
für Herz- und Kreislaufkranke, D-7812 Bad Krozingen (FRG)

Adv. Cardiol., vol. 31, pp. 80–85 (Karger, Basel 1982)

Coronary Bypass Surgery as a Rehabilitative Procedure[1]

Nanette K. Wenger

Emory University School of Medicine, Atlanta, Ga., USA

Rehabilitative goals for the patient after coronary bypass surgery include relief of angina pectoris, improvement in functional status, prolongation of life, and return to work or preillness life-style.

Relief of Symptoms (Angina Pectoris)

Coronary bypass surgery with subsequent medical management is superior to medical management alone in relief of angina pectoris [1–3]. Improvement is due to increased blood supply to the myocardium. After myocardial revascularization, angina is improved in 70–90% of patients; 50–70% have complete pain relief, at least for 3–5 years following surgery.

Improvement in Functional Status

The ejection fraction improves after successful myocardial revascularization and enhancement of function is prominent in segments of myocardium with prior exercise-induced wall motion dysfunction. Even patients whose resting ventricular function does not improve postoperatively have improved overall and regional ventricular function with exercise. This

[1] Adapted from: Cardiac Rehabilitation, vol. 11, No. 3, pp. 1–6; J. med. Ass. Ga. *70:* 457, 1981; and Rehabilitation of the Coronary Patient, Wiley, New York, 2nd ed. (in press), with permission.

change does not occur with unsuccessful revascularization or perioperative infarction [4]. Reversal of exercise-induced hypotension has also been documented postoperatively [3]. It is not known how long this improved myocardial function will be maintained.

The relief of angina with improvement in ventricular function is manifest as improved cardiovascular performance; there is enhancement of aerobic capacity and physical fitness. In addition to this improvement in functional capacity, related primarily to an increase in myocardial oxygen supply, a further increase in exercise capacity occurs after physical conditioning; the major reduction in myocardial oxygen demand occurs during the initial few months of training [5]. Improvement in functional status is also evident as fewer hospital readmissions and less medication use than with medical management alone [6].

Prognostic Features: Enhancement of Survival

Recent data reenforce the improved prognosis after aortocoronary bypass surgery, as well as improved symptoms and function, for appropriately selected patients. Surgery unquestionably improves survival in patients with left main coronary artery obstruction and is requisite if the remaining arterial anatomy and left ventricular function are appropriate [7]. Improved survival is also evident with triple vessel disease and in some patients with double vessel coronary disease, but medical and surgical intervention have comparable survival in patients with single vessel disease.

In evaluating the role of surgery, one must review both morbidity and mortality of the medically-treated illness. Clinical coronary disease is a varying series of events: nonfatal and fatal myocardial infarction, arrhythmias, congestive heart failure, and sudden death; all must be assessed to determine the role of coronary bypass surgery. Delineation of the course of over 1,200 medically-managed patients after cardiac catheterization for chest pain at Duke University [8] provides information about contemporary medical therapy. Patients for whom surgery was elected were excluded; most patients with at least 75% one-, two-, or three-vessel coronary disease were considered operable.

There was a 47% cumulative rate of coronary events during 7 years; 18% of patients had an initial nonfatal infarction, and in 29% the initial event was death. The emphasis on *both* fatal and nonfatal ischemic events deserves reiteration:

'With nonfatal infarction included as an endpoint, the incidence of total ischemic events in several subsets of patients is far greater than is appreciated when survival alone is considered. Nonfatal infarction accounted for approximately one-third of the initial cardiac events afters catheterization in the total group of 1,214 patients. However, in patients with one- or two-vessel disease and normal ventricular function, nonfatal infarction accounted for as much as two-thirds of the initial events. Even in patients with three-vessel disease and normal ventricular function, approximately half of the initial events were nonfatal infarctions. When survival alone is considered in these categories, a significant proportion of the ischemic events are overlooked' [8].

The appropriate question to be asked thus differs in patients with left main, three-, two-, and one-vessel disease, with varying emphasis on fatal and nonfatal acute coronary episodes.

The major predictors of both nonfatal infarction and death in the Duke series [8] were progressive chest pain, the number of diseased vessels, left main coronary stenosis, and left ventricular function. 5-year follow-up of patients with normal ventricular function showed nonfatal initial events in 69, 68, and 50% respectively of patients with one-, two-, and three-vessel disease. Survival from an ischemic event is more likely in patients without left main coronary obstruction and with preserved ventricular function. Increasing obstruction and unstable pain define a poorer outlook, with more patients having a fatal initial event. The 5-year mortality was 27% in the medically-managed patients; they not only had advantages of modern medical therapy, but patients were excluded for whom surgery was elected.

The European Coronary Surgery Study Group report [6] provides contemporary indications for coronary bypass surgery. This study involved over 700 men under age 65, with two or more vessel obstruction of at least 50%, an ejection fraction in excess of 50%; and only mild or moderate angina pectoris. The mortality was one of the lowest ever reported, 92.2%, possibly reflecting selection of patients with modest angina and good ventricular function.

At 3–5 years of follow-up, there was improved survival in the total surgical group, 93.5 vs. 84.1%. With left main disease, the data are 92.9 vs. 61.7%; and with three-vessel disease, 94.9 vs. 84.8%. In addition to a marked decrease in symptoms and drug requirements, improvement in exercise performance occurred in the surgically treated patients. Although no difference in survival was apparent in the total group of patients with two-vessel disease, those with two-vessel disease with proximal LAD obstruction had an 82% survival compared with those without this lesion who had a 96% survival. Therefore, two-vessel disease with proximal LAD involvement must be considered similar to three-vessel disease.

In the 5-year follow-up of 150 patients of *Epstein* et al. [9] with mild angina, annual mortality with three-vessel disease was 5%; patients with good exercise tolerance had a 2.5% annual mortality and with poor exercise tolerance an 11% mortality. Even with mild symptoms, exercise response profoundly affects outcome.

The increasing evidence that surgery prolongs life, however, is an incomplete assessment of the value of surgery. The major problem in most patients with one- and two-vessel disease, and in many with three-vessel disease and intact ventricular function, is *not* mortality but nonfatal ischemic events; thus, the incidence of these events must be compared in medically- and surgically-managed patients.

Vocational and Socioeconomic Concerns

Despite the dramatic symptomatic and functional improvement, rehabilitation, *if* measured by the retention or resumption of gainful employment, has been disappointing. Fewer patients return to work after aortocoronary bypass surgery than after uncomplicated myocardial infarction. *However, insufficient emphasis has been accorded the predominantly nonmedical reasons for failure to return to work.*

After coronary angiography, there was no difference in full-time employment between patients receiving medical and surgical therapy [10]. Increased age at surgery, lower educational level, development of angina postoperatively, prior infarction, and increased physical job requirements influence the decision not to work after surgery [11]. Postoperative clinical results have an insignificant relationship to return to work; improvement in angina or exercise tolerance does not appear to determine employment. Neither is coronary disease severity or completeness of myocardial revascularization of predictive value. This may reflect that few jobs in today's mechanized society demand physical work. This disparity between medical and social outcomes [12] defines that many complex and predominantly *nonmedical* interactions govern return to work.

As after myocardial infarction, the recent work status and the type of occupation (e. g., physical effort involved) after coronary bypass are important factors. Patients who are anxious or depressed, who become symptomatic with effort (i. e., lower functional class), with a lower social class and educational level, those who perceive their illness as job-related, and vocationally disadvantaged patients have a lesser return to work.

Unfortunately, often patients lower on the social class scale, who do physically demanding work, have problems with return to employment; their limited educational skills allow less opportunity for job change.

The major determinant of employment, in both medically- and surgically-treated patients appears to be recent work status; the longer the patient has been unemployed, the less likely the return to work. Since most patients who return to work do so within the 6–10 months after surgery, the attitude of the physician in actively encouraging prompt return to work appears a determining factor. In some reports, a small but significant increase in return to work occurred postoperatively in patients unemployed prior to surgery because of angina.

Other problems are the financial/social/disability/compensation benefits of not returning to work. Many employer and union practices and policies; and governmental and industrial disability, pension, and retirement benefits [12]; encourage patients to remain unemployed. Legislation about employer liability, health care costs, other insurance costs, etc. may also negatively affect the cardiac patient's return to work.

Recent data [13] are slightly more optimistic; although most patients not working preoperatively tended to remain unemployed, some did seek employment, and 22% were employed 4 years after surgery. 90% of patients under age 55 years, employed at the time of surgery, were still employed 4 years postoperatively, comparable to the 93.5% US employment for that age group. In general, the decision not to work was more prevalent among older patients and patients with prior infarction; only 44% of patients aged 60 or more at bypass surgery were employed 4 years later.

Conclusions

In the patient with symptomatic coronary disease, prompt diagnostic evaluation and coronary bypass surgery when appropriate may improve the rehabilitative outcome [14]. Dangers of procrastination include myocardial infarction, cardiac death, and a decreased likelihood of return to work. The physician must, within limits of safety, expeditiously schedule coronary angiography, followed by myocardial revascularization when indicated; and subsequently specifically encourage rapid resumption of an active lifestyle, including return to work.

References

1 Hurst, J. W.; King, S. B.; Logue, R. B.; Hatcher, C. R.; Jones, E. L.; Craver, J. M.; Douglas, J. S.; Franch, R. H.; Dorney, E. R.; Cobbs, B. W.; Robinson, P. H.; Clements, S. D.; Kaplan, J. A.; Bradford, J. M.: Value of coronary bypass surgery. Am. J. Cardiol. *42:* 308 (1978).

2 Zir, L. M.; Dinsmore, R.; Vexerdis, M.; Singh, J. B.; Harthorne, J. W.; Daggett, W. M.: Effects of coronary bypass grafting on resting left ventricular contraction in patients studied 1 to 2 years after operation. Am. J, Cardiol. *44:* 601 (1979).

3 Li, W.; Riggins, R. C. K.; Anderson, R. P.: Reversal of exertional hypotension after coronary bypass grafting. Am. J. Cardiol. *44:* 607 (1979).

4 Bussman, W.-D.; Mayer, V.; Kober, G.; Kaltenbach, M.: Regional ventricular function at rest, during leg raising and physical exercise before and after aortocoronary bypass surgery; in Roskamm, Schmuziger, Coronary heart disease, p. 322 (Springer, New York 1979).

5 Oldridge, N. B.; Nagle, F. J.; Balke, B.; Corliss, R, J,; Kahn, D. R.: Aortocoronary bypass surgery: Effects of surgery and 32 months of physical conditioning on treadmill performance. Archs phys. Med. Rehabil. *59:* 268 (1978).

6 European Coronary Surgery Study Group: Prospective randomized study of coronary artery bypass surgery and stable angina pectoris. Second interim report. Lancet *ii:* 491 (1980).

7 Takaro, T.; Hultgren, H. N.; Lipton, M. J.; Detre, K. M.: The VA cooperative randomized study of surgery for coronary artery occlusive disease. II. Subgroup with significant left main lesions. Circulation *54:* suppl. III, p. 107 (1976).

8 Harris, P. J.; Lee, K. L.; Harrell, F. E.; Behar, B. S.; Rosati, R. A.: Outcome in medically treated coronary artery disease. Ischemic events: nonfatal infarction and deaths. Circulation *62:* 718 (1980).

9 Epstein, S. E.; Kent, K. M.; Goldstein, R. E.; Borer, J. S.; Rosing, D. R.: Strategy for evaluation and surgical treatment of the asymptomatic or mildly symptomatic patients with coronary artery disease. Am. J. Cardiol. *43:* 1015 (1979).

10 Hammermeister, K. E.; DeRouen, T. A.; English, M. T.; Dodge, H. T.: Effect of surgical versus medical therapy on return to work in patients with coronary artery disease. Am. J. Cardiol. *44:* 105 (1979).

11 Barnes, G. K.; Ray, M. J.; Oberman, A,; Kouchoukos, N. T.: Changes in working status of patients following coronary bypass surgery. J. Am. med. Ass. *238:* 1259 (1977).

12 Blumchen, G.; Scharp-Bornhofen, E.; Brand, D.; van den Bergh, C,; Bierk, G.: Clinical results and social implications in patients after coronary bypass surgery; in Roskamm, Schmuziger, Coronary heart disease, p. 375 (Springer, New York 1979).

13 Anderson, A. J.; Barboriak, J. J.; Hoffmann, R. G.; Mullen, D. E.: Retention or resumption of employment after aortocoronary bypass operations. J. Am. med. Ass. *243:* 543 (1980).

14 Crosby, I. K.; Wellons, H. A., Jr.; Martin, R. P.; Schuch, D.; Muller, W. H., Jr.: Employability – a new indication for aneurysmectomy and coronary revascularization. Circulation *62:* suppl. 1, pp. 1–79 (1980).

N. K. Wenger, MD, Emory University School of Medicine,
Thomas K. Glenn Memorial Building, 69 Butler Street, S. E., Atlanta, GA 30303 (USA)

B. Drugs

Adv. Cardiol., vol. 31, pp. 86–89 (Karger, Basel 1982)

Secondary Prevention after Myocardial Infarction

D. G. Julian

British Heart Foundation Professor of Cardiology, University of Newcastle upon Tyne, Freeman Hospital, Newcastle upon Tyne, England

Rehabilitation is a comprehensive concept and involves the restoration of the patient to as normal a life-style and as normal a life-span as possible. There are many approaches to this end, but drug therapy forms an essential component.

For many years, we have depended on nitrates and beta-blocking agents for the control of symptoms in patients with ischaemic heart disease and more recently we have had available the calcium blocking agents. It is becoming increasingly clear that some, if not all, these agents may play a role not only in the relief of symptoms but in prolonging life. Furthermore, there are therapies, such as platelet disaggregating agents and anti-coagulants, that may not improve symptoms but may prevent further catastrophic events, particularly myocardial infarction.

Before considering the variety of drugs which we may use in this context, it is worth while reviewing the known prognostic factors and the ways in which these may be modified.

Those who have developed prognostic indices, particularly in the context of myocardial infarction, have demonstrated that several factors are related to prognosis [1–4]. These include age, sex, number and severity of previous infarctions, severe left ventricular dysfunction and so forth. It is perhaps unfortunate that these prospective studies have concentrated on irreversible prognostic factors, because categorising patients in this way is probably unhelpful in determining which forms of therapy are most likely to be beneficial. Clearly, what we should be attempting to do is to identify specific factors that we can modify with particular forms of therapy. Among such factors, we can consider, for example, the arrhythmias, hypertension, smoking and reversible ischaemia. So far, each of these have been related quite clearly to prognosis, either in the short- or the long-term. We certainly need other prognostic factors, such as those related to clotting, so that we might be able to identify groups of patients who might specifically benefit from anti-platelet or anti-coagulant therapy.

The most convincing evidence of improvement in prognosis by drug therapy has been achieved in the last year by reports on the use of beta-adrenergic blocking drugs. The timolol study from Norway [5] produced almost incontrovertible evidence of the value of this drug in reducing mortality in a period from 12 to 33 months after infarction. It seemed to improve the prognosis in all of 3 risk groups, although perhaps most impressively in a group without previous infarction but with an adverse course during the recent event. One of the most interesting features was the demonstration of the benefit of this drug in preventing sudden, virtually instantaneous, death implying that it is successful in preventing ventricular fibrillation in the absence of fresh myocardial infarction. In November 1981, we have had confirmation of the value of beta-blocking drugs from the propranolol study undertaken in the United States [6]. In this study, it was apparent that in a time period up to 3 years, there was a significant reduction in deaths in patients receiving propranolol of a sufficient degree to convince the organisers that the study should be stopped.

At one time, it seemed as if only one beta-blocking drug might be effective, i.e., timolol, which posed major questions of the mechanism of action. Now, it would seem that we can be more confident that beta-blocking drugs as a whole are effective as, apart from timolol and propranolol, there was suggestive evidence from studies with alprenolol in Sweden [7] and practolol in the United Kingdom and elsewhere [8]. It would, therefore, seem that beta-adrenergic blocking drugs are effective as a group and that no special property is necessary to allow them to prevent death.

It is important to differentiate the use of beta-adrenergic blocking drugs in the long-term after myocardial infarction from their use in the very acute phase. Here the purpose of administering these drugs is different. One hopes that by limiting infarct size, eventual prognosis may be improved. In order to do this, it is clearly necessary to give the drug within the very first hours after infarction. Unfortunately, in the recent metoprolol study from Göteborg [9] the median time of administration was as late as 11 h; this cannot, therefore, be regarded as an early administration study and the benefits achieved may have been due more to an effect similar to that reported in the timolol and propranolol studies referred to previously. The atenolol study by *Sleight* [this volume], and a metoprolol study now being conducted in Belfast, may yield more information on the use of these drugs in the acute phase.

Of course, other strategies are being tested and there are beginning to be encouraging reports in relation to such therapies as nitroprusside and hyaluronidase. The potential use of calcium-blocking drugs and the administration of thrombolytic therapy in the acute phase, clearly may also have an important role in this context.

I think we can be reasonably confident that over the next year or two several new reports will demonstrate that a variety of therapies are beneficial in limiting infarct size and in improving long-term prognosis. Much careful thought must be given to defining populations who may benefit from one or more of these therapies. We cannot assume because a particular drug produces a statistically significant benefit that this drug should be given to all patients. Thus, in the recent metoprolol and propranolol studies, only 2 or 3% of patients were benefited. We should surely be trying to define which patients are likely to be helped and which not by the different varieties of treatment.

References

1 Bigger, J. T.; Heller, C. A.; Wenger, T. L.; Weld, F. M.: Risk stratification after acute myocardial infarction. Am. J. Cardiol. *42:* 202–210 (1978).

2 Kitchin, A. H.; Pocock, S. J.: Prognosis of patients with acute myocardial infarction admitted to a coronary care unit. I. Survival in the hospital. Br. Heart J. *39:* 1163–1166 (1977).

3 Luria, M. H.; Knoke, J. D.; Wachs, J. S.; Luria, M. A.: Survival after recovery from acute myocardial infarction. Am. J. Med. *67:* 7–14 (1979).

4 Norris, R. M.; Caughey, D. E.; Deeming, L. W.; Mercer, C. J.; Scott, P. J.: Coronary prognostic index for predicting survival after recovery from acute myocardial infarction. Lancet *ii:* 484–487 (1970).

5 Norwegian Multicenter Study Group: Timolol-induced reduction in mortality and reinfarction in patients surviving acute myocardial infarction. New Engl. J. Med. *304:* 801–807 (1981).

6 Beta-blocker Heart Attack Study Group: The beta-blocker heart attack trial. J. Am. med. Ass. *246:* 2073–2074 (1981).

7 Wilhelmsson, C.; Vedin, J. A.; Wilhelmsen, L.; Tibblin, G.; Werko, L.: Reduction of sudden deaths after myocardial infarction by treatment with alprenolol. Lancet *ii:* 1157–1159 (1974).
8 Multicentre International Study: Improvement in prognosis of myocardial infarction by long-term beta-adrenoreceptor blockade using practolol. Br. med. J. *iii:* 735–740 (1974).
9 Hjalmarson, A.; Elmfeldt, D.; Herlitz, J.; et al.: Effect on mortality of metoprolol in acute myocardial infarction. Lancet *ii:* 823–827 (1981).

D. G. Julian, MD, British Heart Foundation, University of Newcastle upon Tyne, Freeman Hospital, Newcastle upon Tyne, NE7 7DN (England)

Adv. Cardiol., vol. 31, pp. 90–94 (Karger, Basel 1982)

Beta-Blockade in Acute Myocardial Infarction

P. Sleight

John Radcliffe Hospital, Headington Oxford, University of Oxford, UK

Introduction

Previous trials of beta-adrenoceptor blockade in acute myocardial infarction have been equivocal or negative, despite animal evidence which suggests a possible beneficial effect if given early [2, 3]. In the last 2 or 3 years, the evidence has been more encouraging, probably because of the use of the intravenous route for treatment [6, 11, 13]. The animal evidence suggests that early treatment (within 6h) or pre-treatment is of great importance [3]. We began a trial of intravenous blockade in the first 12 h after the onset of pain of presumed myocardial infarction. A preliminary report on the first 200 patients has been published [13].

We began this trial after we had shown good correlation between ECG and enzyme measures of infarct size [11], and after we had also shown that the evolution of infarction in man was perhaps slower than had been previously emphasised [12]. We began by a double-blind randomised trial of oral Atenolol versus placebo but found that oral treatment might take 6h or more to lower heart rate reliably [10].

Methods

We aimed at a trial size of approximately 400 patients with a preliminary analysis after the first 200 patients. Patients were eligible for randomisation if they met the following criteria: (a) pain thought typical of myocardial infarction present for longer than 30min and beginning less than 12h earlier and (b) no contra-indications to beta-blockade, namely: a history of bronchospasm, hypotension (systolic blood pressure < 100mmHg), bradycardia

(<40/min), obvious heart failure (needing frusemide or digoxin); beta-blocker therapy already instituted; no positive indications for beta-blockers.

The entry ECG was used to allocate patients to two groups, one with 'threatened' infarction showed either no ECG changes or ST changes < 1 mm. The second group included those with more definite changes, i.e. ST change > 2 mm on the 12-lead ECG. Blood samples were drawn at entry and thereafter 4-hourly from an indwelling venous cannula, for measurement of the myocardial component of creatine kinase (CKMB). Cumulative enzyme release was estimated by a modification [4] of the method of *Sobel* et al. [9]. Serial 12-lead ECGs were recorded at entry, on day 3 and on discharge. Infarction was assessed by the R wave score, i.e. the sum of R waves from those leads showing ST or T changes or Q waves. The score was expressed as a percentage of the initial R waves in the same leads.

Those patients judged suitable for the trial were randomised to receive either Atenolol or no Atenolol. We did not use a placebo injection since our preliminary experience suggested that Atenolol usually caused a prompt reduction in heart rate and blood pressure, making a truly blind trial difficult. The treated patients were given 5 mg of Atenolol intravenously slowly over 5 min. If the patient became excessively hypotensive or the heart rate slowed below 40 beats/min the injection was terminated. No further treatment was given. Otherwise the patient received 50 mg orally twice a day for 7 days. The results were analysed by 'intention to treat' regardless of whether the patients did in fact receive the full dose or whether control patients subsequently were given beta-blockade by their physicians. (The general policy in our unit is set by the cardiologists but the prescribing and care in the CCU and in the general ward is done by the admitting team of physicians.)

The study began in the CCU of the John Radcliffe Hospital, Oxford, but was later extended to the Regional Cardiac Centre at the Wythenshawe Hospital, Manchester.

Results

In the initial report [13] we reported a significant reduction in R wave loss and enzyme release in those with 'definite' infarction. The mean reduction in enzyme release was 32% but with wide 95% confidence limits (between 5 and 50% reduction). For this reason the trial was continued. The later analysis has shown a narrowing of the confidence limits to between one sixth and 45% reduction. The ECG data gave very comparable results. In the group with minor acute ECG changes at entry ('threatened' infarction) we found that about 60% subsequently developed raised enzymes (2 times normal) in the control group, whereas only 37% went on to definite infarction in the Atenolol group.

Complications

We had of course been worried whether acute intravenous beta-blockade early in myocardial infarction would precipitate heart failure. We had been reassured on this point by the preliminary reports on this point from *Hjalmarson* et al. [1] in Gothenberg, and our own subsequent experience confirmed this. On the contrary, heart failure during the hospital stay, the total dose of diuretics, and the need for diuretics and/or digoxin on discharge were significantly less in the beta-blocked group [13]. Hypotension and bradycardia were more common in the Atenolol group but only rarely posed a problem. Treatment was limited to atropine in the majority of cases. Inotropic agents were used in only 5 patients (3 Atenolol, 2 control) in the first 200 patients. Arrythmias were more common in the control group. A more detailed analysis of the first 24h of taped ECGs in 100 consecutive patients by *Rossi* et al. [8] in my department has shown significantly fewer R-on-T ectopics in the Atenolol group.

Mortality

The trial was not intended to study mortality since it seemed that we would be unlikely to see any significant difference in the small number of deaths we expected. It was encouraging that in the preliminary report we found fewer deaths in the Atenolol group (4 vs. 9) and fewer in the hospital deaths or non fatal cardiac arrests (5 vs. 14).

Preliminary analysis of our final results in this trial [unpublished] shows a significant ($p = < 0.02$) reduction in mortality at 7 days.

Discussion

This study has suggested that acute intravenous beta-blockade can be useful in carefully selected patients early in the development of acute myocardial infarction. Why has this trial been more encouraging than earlier trials? We feel several reasons may have been responsible. First, the patients were treated much earlier than in previous trials; 75% of our patients were treated within 6h of the onset of pain. Second, intravenous therapy produces an effect upon rate-pressure product within minutes [7]. Third, the trial was of adequate size to demonstrate the effect. We should emphasise that care should be taken to exclude patients may need atropine and/or inotropic agents to reverse excessive hypotension and bradycardia. For these reasons we would not recommend indiscriminate or community use of this therapy unless the physician was experienced with the drug and willing and able to stay with the patient some time.

Controlled randomised evaluation of its use by primary care physicians would seem a high priority, in order to achieve the earliest treatment.

We have begun a large multicentre randomised study to examine mortality experience in greater detail.

Since this trial was first reported, two new and important trials have been published. The Norwegian trial of Timolol [5] has justly received considerable praise for its size and quality. This trial was a late-entry trial in those who had survived a myocardial infarction and showed a very favourable effect of Timolol in reducing sudden death. The Swedish Metoprolol trial [1] gave initial acute intravenous treatment but followed this with 3-month oral treatment with placebo or Metoprolol. There was a significant reduction of mortality and of infarct size, but most of this mortality reduction occurred after the first 10 days; the mortality curves were very similar to the Timolol study. It may be that this lack of a very early effect (in contrast to our study) is due to the fact that the intravenous therapy was given rather late (a mean of 11.3h after the onset of pain compared with our median of 4h).

These two latest trials together with our Atenolol study do make it very probable that the favourable results are due to beta-blockade, per se, and not to any other property of the drugs, such as membrane stabilisation or cardioselectivity. They also suggest that there is now sufficient evidence that beta-blockade favourably influences survival after a myocardial infarction. I do not think we yet have enough evidence to know reliably whether very early intravenous beta-blockade will reduce mortality further. Our own and the Swedish results are encouraging.

We are at present conducting a large randomised trial in 8,000–10,000 patients in over 100 centres, about half of which are in the UK and half in many other different countries.

References

1 Hjalmarson, A.; Elmfeldt, D.; Herlitz, J.; Holmberg, S.; Maler, I.; Nyberg, G.; Ryden, L.; Swedberg, K.; Vedin, A.; Waagstein, F.; Waldenstrom, A.; Waldenstrom, J.; Wedel, H.; Wilhelmsen, L.; Wilhelmsson, C.: Effect on mortality of metoprolol in acute myocardial infarction. A Double-blind randomised trial. Lancet *ii:* 823–827 (1981).

2 Jennings, R. B.; Reimer, K. A.: Salvage of ischaemic myocardium. Med. Conc. cardiovasc. Dis. *43:* 125–130 (1974).

3 Miura, N.; Thomas, R.; Ganz, W.; Sokol, T.; Shell, W. E.; Toshimitsu, T.; Kwan, A. C.; Singh, B. N.: The effect of delay in propranolol administration of reduction of myocardial infarct size after experimental coronary artery occlusion in dogs. Circulation *59:* 1148 (1979).

4 Norris, R. M.; Whitlock, R. M. L.; Barratt-Boyes, C.; Small, C. W.: Clinical measurement of myocardial infarct size: modification of a method for the estimation of creatine phosphokinase release after myocardial infarction. Circulation *51:* 614–620 (1975).

5 The Norwegian Multicentre Study Group. Timolol-induced reduction in mortality and reinfarction in patients surviving acute myocardial infarction. New Engl. J. Med. *304:* 801–807 (1981).

6 Peter, T.; Norris, R. M.; Clarke, E. D.; Heng, M. K.; Singh, B. M.; Williams, B.; Howell, D. R.; Ambler, P. K.: Reduction of enzyme levels by propranolol after acute myocardial infarction. Circulation *57:* 1091–1095 (1978).

7 Ramsdale, D. R.; Farragher, E. B.; Bennett, D. H.; Bray, C.; Ward, C.; Cruickshank, J. M.; Yusuf, S.; Sleight, P.: Pain relief in acute myocardial infarction by intra-venous Atenolol. Am. Heart J. (in press, 1981).

8 Rossi, P. R. F.; Yusuf, S.; Ramsdale, D.; Peto, R.; Furze, L.; Bennett, D.; Bray, C.; Sleight, P.: Reduction in R-on-T ectopics and rate of ventricular tachycardia by early intravenous beta blockade in acute myocardial infarction. Br. Heart J. (in press, 1981).

9 Sobel, B. E.; Bresnahan, G. F.; Shell, W. E.; Yoder, R. D.: Estimation of infarct size in man and its relation to prognosis. Circulation *46:* 640–648 (1972).

10 Yusuf, S.: Beta blockade in acute myocardial infarction; D. Phil. thesis Oxford (1980).

11 Yusuf, S.; Lopez, R.; Maddison, A.; Maw, P.; Ray, N.; McMillian, S.; Sleight, P.: Value of electrocardiogram in predicting and estimating infarct size in man. Br. Heart J. *42:* 286–293 (1979).

12 Yusuf, S.; Lopez, R.; Maddison, A.; Sleight, P.: Electrocardiographic and enzyme evolution of infarct size in man. Circulation *57/58:* suppl. II, p. 172 (1978).

13 Yusuf, S.; Ramsdale, D.; Peto, R.; Furse, L.; Bennett, D.; Bray, C.; Sleight, P.: Early intravenous Atenolol treatment in suspect acute myocardial infarction. Preliminary report of a randomised trial. Lancet *ii:* 273–276 (1980).

Prof. P. Sleight, John Radcliffe Hospital, University of Oxford,
Headington, Oxford OX3 9DU (UK)

Adv. Cardiol., vol. 31, pp. 95–97 (Karger, Basel 1982)

Prevention of Ischaemic Heart Disease in the Hypertensive Patient

Michael Thomas

Midhurst Medical Research Institute, Midhurst, West Sussex, UK

There is a progressive tendency for arterial pressure to rise with advancing age in western countries. Because this seems 'natural' there has been an inclination to assess blood pressure as normal or high in relation to the average for a particular age. There is increasing evidence to support a less conventional view that arterial pressure levels higher than those commonly found in the second decade of life may be harmful both as regards illness in later life and ultimate life expectancy. This hypothesis follows earlier work in the treatment of hypertension dictated by the occurrence of cerebral complications, including stroke, and also by renal failure [1]. The success in largely eliminating stroke and renal failure as causes of death in well-controlled hypertensives is now well known. Left-ventricular failure figured in the arguments for treating high arterial pressure but for the most part cardiac matters were not in the forefront. The natural history of treated hypertensives is now dominated by heart complications and cardiac death.

Hypertension affects the heart primarily in two major ways – through the heart muscle and the coronary arteries. Coronary artery disease secondarily further involves the heart muscle at a later stage.

The progress of systemic artery systolic pressure in western men is broadly represented by an increase from 120 mm Hg in the second decade of life to 160 mm Hg or above in the sixth or seventh decade [2]. Elevation of the left-ventricular pressure to progressively higher levels involves the heart in the need to generate more contractile force. As a secondary consequence, hypertrophy of the left-ventricular muscle takes place. The muscle thickening proceeds to a very variable degree in individuals but in general begins to be evident as electrocardiographic changes around systolic pressures of 150 mm Hg. The thickened myocardium sometimes associated with an increased ventricular diastolic pressure leads to an abnormal coronary vascular behaviour when the heart fluctuates between conditions of different loading. The blood flow to the endocardium can become compromised under certain mechanical conditions even in the absence of main stem coronary artery disease [3]. High aortic blood pressure is 'experienced' by the coronary arterial wall over many years. Secondary changes follow. Arteries become thickened, and it is thought from epidemiological studies in hypertensives, that the severity and rapidity of atherosclerotic generation becomes more marked. Quantified relationships are not available but it would also seem likely from epidemiological studies that smoking has an important additive, or multiplicatory, adverse influence on atheromatous degeneration.

It is easily seen that the hypertensive heart determines its own fate by requiring progressively more myocardial blood flow to satisfy the need for greater mechanical work, and at the same time, becoming less and less able to supply such flow on demand because of coronary atherosclerosis and defects in endocardial flow dynamics. The importance of myocardial ischaemia and infarction as the dominant cause of death in treated western hypertensives is now well documented.

Hypertensive therapy needs a cardiac orientation if this last problem is to be overcome. It is important that the systolic load conferred on the heart is prevented at an early stage. Treatment should begin at quite low levels of hypertension, for example 150/90 mm Hg. Inescapably this will imply that many individuals will take tablets for very many years. If arterial pressure is prevented from rising to any great degree, any secondary effect of hypertension per se on arterial walls will be minimised and main stem arterial disease should progress less rapidly. Unfortunately, this desirable state of affairs is most unlikely to be attained on a wide scale and we have to do our best with hearts that have already suffered to a moderate degree.

Sudden death is usually associated with two or three severe coronary artery stenoses [4]. In the hypertrophic left ventricle supplied by atheromatous coronary arteries the dangerous haemodynamic variations include rapid rise in heart rate, tension time index and ventricular diastolic pressure. These changes compromise the heart by together increasing the ratio of myocardial tension work to the available oxygen supply, especially in the endocardium. At a certain stage in the natural history of high blood pressure, the heart becomes very vulnerable to local and global ischaemia. Prevention of abrupt increase in these haemodynamic parameters protects the heart against ischaemia. 'Tailor-made' for such prevention is a beta-blocking drug. It has been shown that such agents curtail the oxygen requirement of the heart by governing both heart rate and tension-time index. Through limitation of heart frequency and a rise in left-ventricular diastolic pressure on load, endocardial perfusion is favoured. Overall myocardial oxygen requirement in the presence of beta-blockade is governed by rate and tension-time index reduction and limitation [5]. These mechanisms are probably sufficient to explain the symptomatic improvement in hypertensive patients with angina pectoris following treatment with beta-blockade.

One would expect that restricting the ventricular pressure x time integral to the range found in youth would confer security against acute hypertensive heart failure. While the heart is able to operate within the confines of adequate myocardial blood flow there should also be security against acute myocardial ischaemia. Whether this is the case in practice has been the subject of clinical trial. There is a certain amount of evidence in favour of this hypothesis from the studies of *Lambert* [6], *Stewart* [7], and *Berglund* et al. [8] who have all indicated fewer serious ischaemic cardiac events in hypertensive patients treated by beta-blocking agents. There is at present little or no evidence to argue against such a policy.

References

1 Veterans Administration Cooperative Study Group on Antihypertensive Agents. J. Am. med. Ass. *213:* 1143 (1970).

2 Peart, W. S.: Concepts in hypertension. The Croonian Lecture 1979. Il R. Coll. Physns Lond. *14:* 141–152 (1980).

3 Rembert, J. C.; Kleinman, L. H.; Fedor, J. M.; Wechsler, A. S.; Greenfield, J. C.: Myocardial blood flow distribution in concentric left ventricular hypertrophy. J. clin. Invest. *62:* 379–386 (1978).

4 Davies, M. J.: Pathological view of sudden cardiac death. Br. Heart J. *45:* 88–96 (1981).

5 Thomas, M.; Gabe, I. T.; Kimber, H.; Mills, C. J.; Sweeting, T. J.: Does beta-blockade directly reduce myocardial oxygen consumption? Cardiovasc. Res. *15:* 254–261 (1981).

6 Lambert, D. M. D.: Hypertension and myocardial infarction. Br. med. J. *iii:* 685 (1974).

7 Steward, I. McD. G.: Compared incidence of first myocardial infarction in hypertensive patients under treatment containing propranolol or excluding beta-receptor blockade. Clin. Sci. mol. Med. *51:* 509S–511S (1976).

8 Berglund, G.; Wilhelmsen, L.; Sannerstedt, R.; Hansson, L.; Andersson, O.; Silvertsson, R.; Wedel, H.; Wikstrand, J.: Coronary heart disease after treatment of hypertension. Lancet *i:* 1–5 (1978).

M. Thomas, MD, The Midhurst Medical Research Institute, Midhurst, West Sussex (UK)

Adv. Cardiol., vol. 31, pp. 98–101 (Karger, Basel 1982)

Anticoagulants and Platelet-Active Agents in the Secondary Prevention of Coronary Artery Disease

W. G. Van Aken

Department of Internal Medicine, University Hospital 'Wilhelmina Gasthuis', and Central Laboratory of the Netherlands Red Cross Blood Transfusion Service, Amsterdam, The Netherlands

Introduction

Acute myocardial infarction occurs predominantly in patients with some degree of coronary artery disease. Such affected vessels are prone to develop arterial thrombosis either before infarction or as a secondary phenomenon, relatively late after infarction. Several post mortem studies and clinicopathologic correlations have shown a strong association between acute coronary occlusion and regional myocardial infarcts.

Clinical and experimental evidence suggests that arterial thrombosis, emboli and substances released from platelets may mediate a series of acute vascular events including myocardial infarction. The interaction between platelets and subendothelial vascular structures initiates the formation of a platelet thrombus. In addition, the generation of thrombin after vessel injury may both augment platelet reactivity and lead to fibrin formation. In an attempt to prevent thromboemboli in the coronary artery system, both platelet-active agents and anticoagulants have been used in several clinical trials. In this report, only results of those clinical studies are discussed that have used recurrent myocardial infarction and mortality as clinical end-point.

Anticoagulants

Most of the studies on oral anticoagulants in the prevention of myocardial infarction have been performed before 1970. Although anticoagulants reduced mortality to a statistically significant degree in a few of these studies, failures in trial design and in control of anticoagulant effect precluded definite conclusions about efficacy [1]. Thus, the indications for oral anticoagulants in acute myocardial infarction are still arbitrary.

In the Netherlands, two double-blind trials, performed in 1967–1969, indicated that long-term anticoagulant therapy is effective in reducing recurrent infarction [2, 3]. Since then a large number of patients with myocardial infarction received this therapy which is controlled by special centres distributed all over the country. To determine its efficacy in patients over 60 years of age, in whom haemorrhagic side effects may outweigh the potentially favourable effects, a randomised double-blind multicentre trial in the Netherlands has been recently completed [4]. Half of the patients who had been on anticoagulants since their first myocardial infarction received placebos instead of anticoagulants, whereas the others continued anticoagulant therapy. It was shown that continuation of intensive and stable anticoagulant therapy significantly reduced the risk of recurrent myocardial infarction and mortality. Although the number of bleeding episodes was greater in the patients receiving anticoagulants, the incidence of both intracranial events and fatal extracranial haemorrhages was not different in the two groups. Definite conclusions as to the effects of anticoagulant treatment in acute myocardial infarction cannot be drawn from this study. However, the results demonstrated that adequate control of hypocoagulability is an absolute requirement during the follow-up.

Further studies are required to establish if well-controlled anticoagulant treatment, when started shortly following myocardial infarction is beneficial and if in certain categories this effect is more (or less) pronounced. In the meantime, anticoagulants can be recommended in patients with large infarctions, congestive heart failure, atrial fibrillation, ventricular aneurysms and complications requiring prolonged bed-rest.

Platelet-Active Agents

Acetylsalicylic acid (aspirin), dipyridamole (Persantin) and sulfinpyrazone (Anturane), either alone or in combination, have been tested in several large, randomized, double-blind multicentre trials in patients who survived after the first myocardial infarction [for a review, see ref. 5]. It should be noted that the design of these trials was not uniform. For instance, the time from myocardial infarction to enrolment and the dosage of aspirin varied considerably across these studies. Furthermore, in some studies, patients were withdrawn for some reason (e. g. side effects) but were not included in the analysis, which may bias the results.

The initial studies with aspirin found trends in mortality favourable to aspirin but statistical significance was not reached.

In the recently completed Aspirin Myocardial Infarction Study (AMIS) [6], no benefit was derived from aspirin in terms of mortality although the incidence of recurrent, non-fatal myocardial infarction was lower in the aspirin-treated group (6.3%) than in the placebo group (8.1%). The benefit is, however, outbalanced by the increased incidence of side effects (23.7% vs. 14.9%) in the aspirin group. The authors of AMIS conclude that aspirin is not recommended for routine use in patients who have survived myocardial infarction. To this conclusion may be added: 'at least at the dosage used', since in vitro and animal studies have demonstrated that aspirin, by acetylating cyclo-oxygenase, not only inhibits platelet aggregation, but may also decrease the synthesis of prostacyclin by the vascular wall. By adjusting (lowering) the dosage of aspirin it may be possible to inhibit platelet function without affecting prostaglandin synthesis by vascular cells.

In the Persantin Aspirin Reinfarction Study (PARIS) [7] patients were randomized into three groups: Persantin plus aspirin, aspirin alone and placebo. Again, no effect on total mortality in the whole group was observed but those patients who were admitted within 6 months of infarction showed a 50% reduction in mortality when treated with either aspirin or Persantin aspirin. In addition, coronary mortality and non-fatal myocardial infarction after 1 year were 50% lower in the Persantin-aspirin group than in the placebo group, whereas the difference compared with the aspirin-treated group was less clear. PARIS I does not provide a definite answer about the effect of Persantin on cardiac mortality, but hopefully Paris II will demonstrate whether such a treatment may influence mortality if initiated early after myocardial infarction.

The most positive study reported thus far, the Anturane Reinfarction Trial (ART) [8], demonstrated a 74% reduction in sudden death in sulfinpyrazone-treated patients during the first 6 months of follow-up. It should be noted that all patients entered this study between 25 and 35 days after myocardial infarction, whereas in the AMIS and PARIS trials only a small proportion of the patients were included soon after their infarction. There was, however, no significant decrease in the number of reinfarctions in patients receiving sulfinpyrazone. This study has been severely critized for reasons of data analysis and definitions. One should await the results of a re-analysis, which is being performed at the moment, before conclusions can be drawn.

Thus definite recommendations about the indications for platelet-active agents in patients with coronary artery disease cannot be given for the time being. It would seem that the combination of Persantin and aspirin reduces coronary events. However, a decrease of mortality has not yet been observed.

References

1 Gifford, R. H.; Feinstein, A. R.: A critique of methodology in studies of anticoagulant therapy for acute myocardial infarction. New Engl. J. Med. *280:* 351–357 (1969).

2 Loeliger, E. A.; Hensen, A.; Kroes, F.: A double-blind trial of long-term anticoagulant treatment after myocardial infarction. Acta med. scand. *182:* 549–566 (1967).

3 Meuwissen, O. J. A. T.; Vervoorn, A. C.; Cohen, O.: Double-blind trial of long-term anticoagulant treatment after myocardial infarction. Acta med. scand. *186:* 361–368 (1969).

4 Report of the Sixty Plus Reinfarction Study Research Group: A double-blind trial to assess long-term oral anticoagulant therapy in elderly patients after myocardial infarction. Lancet *iii:* 989–994 (1980).

5 Genton, E.: A perspective on platelet-suppressant drug treatment in coronary artery and cerebrovascular disease. Circulation *62:* suppl. V, pp. 111–121 (1980).

6 Aspirin Myocardial Infarction Study Research Group: A randomized, controlled trial of aspirin in persons recovered from myocardial infarction. J. Am. med. Ass. *243:* 661–669 (1980).

7 The Persantin-Aspirin Reinfarction Study Research Group. Persantine and aspirin in coronary heart disease. Circulation *62:* 449–461 (1980).

8 The Anturane Reinfarction Trial Research Group: Sulfinpyrazone in the prevention of sudden death upon myocardial infarction. New Engl. J. Med. *302:* 250–255 (1980).

Dr. W. G. Van Aken, Central Laboratory of the Netherlands Red Cross Blood Transfusion Service, Plesmanlaan 125, NL-1066 CX Amsterdam (The Netherlands)

C. Rehabilitation Programs

Adv. Cardiol., vol. 31, pp. 102–106 (Karger, Basel 1982)

Present and Future of Cardiac Rehabilitation

H. Denolin

Laboratoire de recherches cardiologiques, Université Libre de Bruxelles, Hôpital Saint Pierre, Bruxelles, Belgique

Over the past 30 years, cardiology has witnessed astonishing developments: new methods of investigation, new drugs, development of cardiac surgery. Epidemiology has improved our knowledge of the natural history of cardiac disease and, hopefully, the on-going prevention trials will yield favorable results. Nevertheless, in spite of a decrease in mortality in some countries, cardiac diseases still remain the primary cause of mortality and morbidity in the technically developed world. This means that all possible measures should be taken to reduce to a minimum the consequences of chronic cardiopathies: this is the task of *rehabilitation* which aims to limit as much as possible the physiological, social and psychological consequences of the chronic diseases affecting heart and vessels.

A definition of rehabilitation was given by the European Office of WHO [1] in 1969, which is still complete and valid:

'The rehabilitation of cardiac patients can be defined as the sum of activities required to ensure them the best possible physical, mental and social conditions so that they may, by their own efforts, resume as normal a place as possible in the life of the community.'

'Rehabilitation should take place at an early stage and be continuous. The physician must bear it in mind from his very first contact with the patient and not lose sight of it in any of the phases of treatment or supervision. Every aspect of the patient must be taken into account in rehabilitation, including his physiological, clinical psychological and social problems. Lastly, rehabilitation cannot be regarded as an isolated form of therapy, but must be integrated with the whole treatment of which it constitutes only one facet.'

In the first half of this century, it was a tradition to impose, after a myocardial infarction, prolonged bed rest of at least 6 weeks, and most of the patients became, after a coronary event, definitively invalid. It was in 1944 that *Levine,* and later *Levine and Lown,* stressed the beneficial effect and the absence of risk of rest in a chair from the end of the first week after the accident. Progressively, the concept of early mobilization was developed, and the usefulness of a physical training was accepted. Today, patiens are mobilized, when there are no contraindications, 1 or 2 days after a myocardial infarction, and leave the hospital after 10–15 days. Some of them are intensively trained after 6–8 weeks. In our center, early testing is now advocated before leaving the hospital. The physiological and clinical benefits of these new attitudes are well known.

Unfortunately, for many years only the physiological aspects of rehabilitation have been taken into consideration; the psychological approach and the social problems took much longer to make progress. More recently, secondary prevention was included in rehabilitation programmes. New drugs and coronary surgery were also beneficial in the scope of rehabilitation of the coronary patient.

Today we arrive at a complete and comprehensive programme of rehabilitation after myocardial infarction, which responds to the WHO definition, which is generally accepted in spite of large differences in practical application. It is generally agreed that early mobilization, physical exercise, functional evaluation, psycho-social approach, return to work and secondary prevention are of equal importance: these attitudes are without danger and are, at least in *short time,* of tremendous benefit as compared with the attitudes of the past. The physical condition of the patient is increased, the unfavorable effects of psychological stress are decreased, patients return to work earlier and more easily, etc. We have now sufficient data in the literature to accept the usefulness of our present attitude; but we should accept the idea that, in many aspects, the scientific basis of this new approach remains fragile and that in many areas we do not yet know the optimal attitude. The changes in the rehabilitation programme that we accept today are only trends, and more research is needed to improve our knowledge and to decrease the consequences of a coronary attack as much as possible. The present attitude should not become a definite rule or a dogma before a careful and permanent analysis of our rehabilitation programme has been made.

In Europe, as a result of several years preparatory work, a WHO coordinated study on rehabilitation and comprehensive secondary prevention was designed. This study was aimed at assessing the effectiveness of comprehensive rehabilitation in reducing recurrent myocardial infarction and cardiovascular mortality. Patients under the age of 65 with definite myocardial infarction, treated in hospital, were admitted to the study. The intervention measures were to be applied according to the best knowledge in each individual center. The follow-up period was 3 years. The main end-points were death and morbidity. Physical working capacity, changes in the quality of life and reduction of risk factors were used as additional criteria. The total number of patients (3118), recruted from 19 European centers, were divided in two groups by randomization [2, 3].

Considering the end-points, the pooling of all the data is quite impossible, related to local attitudes and other reasons. If we consider the 17 centers with a sufficient number of patients in the treated and control groups, 13 have mortality experience which favors the rehabilitation group. The difference in reinfarction in the two groups is not significant. There were big intercenter differences in return to work. In most of the centers, the physical capacity is improved. The local differences in results are very important, and demonstrate how difficult the long-term evaluation is.

In the group of patients in Finland for the WHO study, 375 patients were included. The total mortality and the cardiac mortality are lower in the intervention group: these data suggest that patients with myocardial infarction would benefit from an organized comprehensive rehabilitation [3]. But, in one of the Belgian groups, the mortality in the control group was 0% after 3 years, against 6% in the rehabilitation group. This again demonstrates the difficulties of such a study, related to the insufficent number of patients and the local differences in methodology, etc.

In the US, the National Exercise and Heart Disease Project has evaluated the effects of regularly performed, medically prescribed exercise in male survivors of myocardial infarction, who where assigned by randomization to either an exercise group or a nontreated group. This trial was effective in inducing a physiologic training effect, at least for a short time.

The conclusions are that a 37% reduction in mortality was observed in the exercise group, which re-enforces the concept of a beneficial effect of exercise in patients with coronary disease. There is no suggestion of benefit from the programme to cardiovascular morbidity. The number of patients is low (651), and some of them entered the programme 36 months after the myocardial infarction [4].

The results of the Ontario Exercise Heart Collaborative Study are not yet known. But from preliminary data, it appears that, for a total number of

751 patients divided in to 2 groups and submitted to high or low intensity exercise, the drop-out was very high in both groups and the rate of recurrence was not significantly different between the groups [5].

The difficulties in the interpretation of all these data are numerous: low number of subjects, short follow-up, low compliance to the programme, drop-out, mode of selection in the different centers and probably the very important problem of 'drop-in' or contamination of the control group by the new therapeutic attitudes.

A good conclusion is presented by *Shephard* [5]: 'Pessimists might conclude that a controlled study to determine the influence of exercise upon the rate of reinfarction is logistically impossible... optimists might attempt to meet the requirements of large groups by pooling data from various controlled studies, ignoring obvious differences of philosophy and protocol.'

In fact, whole rehabilitation programmes appear to provide many objections and they have failed to show clearly whether survival can be improved.

In conclusion: important changes in the therapeutic approach to myocardial infarction have been made during the last 2 decades. The current attitudes have modified the way of life and the perspectives of our patients: most of them reintegrate easily into family and professional life, and even if it is not ascertained that their life expectations are improved, the quality of their life is. The social and economical benefits are of importance.

But we have to accept that, in spite of excellent results in a short time, the changes in our therapeutic attitudes are based on empiricism, and we cannot say that our actual attitudes are optimal. We need more research for all the parts of the programme, based on a scientific evaluation: intensity and duration of the training programme should be better defined, probably on a more individual basis, through a better selection of the patients, utilizing the possibilities of the new noninvasive methods; psychological problems should be better understood and better treated; prescription of vocational and leisure time activity and their long-term effects should be studied; results of secondary prevention should be clarified, etc.

Finally, the social organization needs better evaluation, and more and difficult research on the effects of a comprehensive programme on the progress of the disease and on the quality of life are needed. The present is characterized by a better quality of life after myocardial infarction, and we have to hope that the future will also be characterized by a better quantity of life.

The task for the future is a permanent critical and scientific control of our present attitudes.

References

1 WHO, Regional Office for Europe: The rehabilitation of patients with cardiovascular disease. Report of a seminar. EURO 0381 (1969).
2 WHO, Europe Office: Study of the effects of rehabilitation and comprehensive secondary prevention in patients after acute myocardial infarction (to be published).
3 Kallio, V.: Evaluation of earlier studies: Europe; in Cohen, et al., Physical conditioning and cardiovascular rehabilitation (Wiley, New York 1981).
4 Tristani, F. E.: National intervention trials and their descendants; in Long, Prevention and rehabilitation in ischemic heart disease (William Wilkins, Baltimore 1980).
5 Shepard, R. J.: Evaluation of earlier studies: Canada; in Cohen, et al., Physical conditioning and cardiovascular rehabilitation (Wiley, New York 1981).

Prof. H. Denolin, MD, 178, Avenue Winston Churchill, B–1180 Bruxelles (Belgium)

Adv. Cardiol., vol. 31, pp. 107–111 (Karger, Basel 1982)

Rehabilitation and Secondary Prevention of Patients after Acute Myocardial Infarction

WHO Collaborative Study

G. Lamm, H. Denolin, D. Dorossiev, Z. Pisa
World Health Organization, Copenhagen, Denmark

Background

In spite of the widespread acceptance of the usefulness of early mobilization and subsequent relatively early physical training after acute myocardial infarction (AMI), the question whether this new approach reduces recurrences and prolongs life was still unanswered in the late sixties. 23 European centres and one in Israel expressed interest in launching a long-term multicentre study to elucidate this problem. The European Office of WHO acted as coordinator from the very beginning. During the first orientation meetings several facts became clear.

(1) A study on the effects of regular physical exercise alone was neither feasible, nor tenable in view of the recent knowledge in secondary prevention.

(2) Large differences between centres, mainly in socioeconomic and legislative conditions, but also in other aspects demanded that the evaluation of the study should be kept at the national level and only trends should be pooled.

(3) The study would be much more a public health trial of the systematic application of up-to-date concepts in rehabilitation and secondary prevention, than a purely scientific multicentre trial.

Bearing these facts in mind, the protocol of a randomized, controlled trial was developed with as much standardization of the methods and criteria as possible. Recurrent AMI and cardiovascular disease (CVD) mortality were the primary endpoints of the study, but softer endpoints, such as return to work, psychosocial and vocational readjustment were also monitored.

Table I. Significant baseline differences between rehabilitation and control groups (percentages)

Characteristics	Rehabilitation group	Control group
Intermittent claudication, %	6.6	9.9
Arterial hypertension, %	21.3	24.7
NYHA severity class I, %	73.8	72.4
NYHA severity class III–IV, %	2.5	4.5
Present smokers, %	65.2	68.1
Congestive heart failure, %	21.0	25.1
Resting AP, %	16.3	23.5
Effort AP, %	22.7	27.8
Age, years	52.3	53.5

NYHA = New York Heart Association; AP = Angina pectoris.

Men below the age of 65 years were randomly allocated to the intervention and control groups on the 28th day after their qualifying AMI. Controls were treated according the prevailing methods in each centre. Intervention – executed throughout by the research-team – comprised physical exercise, anti-smoking and dietary advice, blood pressure and weight control and psychological and vocational assistance when needed.

These measures were applied throughout the 3 years of the study. Initial standardized examination and yearly follow-up was obligatory for both groups. Enrolment started in 1973 and ended in 1975 and the follow-up period was closed by the end of 1978.

Of the 24 original centres only 17 remained for the final evaluation. Accordingly, from the 3,184 enrolled patients, only 2,056 could be considered for evaluation.

Results

Due to different systems of randomization applied in the various centres, the rehabilitation and control groups were not fully comparable in a number of centres at the beginning. When data from all centres were pooled (table I) these differences were all in favour of the rehabilitation group. They were younger, had less severe disease and lower risk factor levels than the control group. From the comparison of reported intervention measures, it emerged that intensity of intervention also differed between centres.

Table II. Percentage of death from all causes after 3 years in the rehabilitation and control groups by centre

Centre code	Death, %		Significance of difference
	rehabilitation group	control group	
01	16.6	27.1	
02	18.2	3.6	$p < 0.01$
03	11.9	15.0	
04	20.8	17.2	
05	19.4	20.0	
08	22.4	30.8	
09	19.0	31.2	$p < 0.054$
15	21.5	25.0	
19	10.7	10.9	
20	5.7	15.6	$p < 0.01$
21	16.1	20.5	
22	2.6	16.9	$p < 0.053$
23	11.0	9.8	
31	8.6	7.0	
51	17.6	21.5	
53	21.5	12.1	
54	7.7	16.7	

The protocol of the study was changed after the first year, by making the 3- and 6-month follow-up visits optional instead of obligatory. All these rendered the evaluation even more difficult than was anticipated.

For the sake of brevity, only the table on total mortality is shown (table II). CVD contributed to the bulk of mortality anyhow – as expected. Significant difference between the rehabilitation and control group was observed in only two centres, although in the opposite direction. Two other centres came close to a significant difference – both in favour of the intervention group.

11 of the 17 centres have mortality experience favouring the rehabilitation group, while in 4 centres mortality was higher in the rehabilitation group. In 2 centres no difference could be observed.

The 2 centres which contributed the largest number of patients to the study (centre 20: 405 cases; centre 53: 294 cases) showed contradictory results. While in centre 20 was a highly significant benefit in terms of mortality for rehabilitation, in centre 53 there were more deaths in that group, although not significantly more.

Non-fatal re-infarctions were less common in the rehabilitation group in 8 centres, while in the remaining 9 the opposite was true. Significant difference was found only in 1 centre and this was in the wrong direction. While these results at 3 years are inconsistent, attention should be paid to the fact that in the first 3 months after AMI there were no non-fatal re-infarctions in the control group in 12 centres, but such events occurred in the rehabilitation group in 11 out of the 17 centres. However, the difference in individual centres was again not significant.

Return to work was higher in the rehabilitation group than in the control in 15 of the 17 centres. However, significant differences were found in only 5 centres. The very large intercentre differences in return to work after 1 year (from 47 to 96%) reflect differences in the social system and legislation. Multivariate analysis of the results was attempted in order to take into account baseline differences between the two groups. Due to the small number of patients in many centres this approach turned out to be unfeasible.

Conclusion

In conclusion it can be stated that the study failed to give an unequivocal answer to the main questions it asked. Neither mortality nor morbidity, nor the softer endpoints like return to work demonstrated consistent benefits for systematic rehabilitation and secondary prevention, as applied in this study.

Thorough analysis of the results tends to show three main reasons for this failure:

(1) The intervention measures were not applied with vigour and consistency as laid down in the protocol.

(2) Information on the habitual measures applied to the control group was insufficient, but it seems that the difference in intervention between the two groups was too small.

(3) Large intercentre differences made it impossible to pool the data for analysis, while the small number of patients in many centres led to the failure to detect any statistically significant differences.

As similar unequivocal results were found in other large collaborative studies, one is inclined to conclude that answers to the still open questions in rehabilitation should be sought for in small, tightly controlled specific studies in well-selected patients and not in large multicentre trials.

The lack of any serious adverse effects from the applied measures is in itself a reassuring finding. Any safe approach which produces less psychological and social cripples and more readjusted patients, is a worthwhile exercise – even if we cannot yet measure its benefits. And perhaps one needs less sophistication and more common sense to achieve this.

Dr. G. Lamm, Regional Officer, World Health Organization,
8 Sherfigwvej, DK-2100 Copenhagen (Denmark)

Adv. Cardiol., vol. 31, pp. 112–119 (Karger, Basel 1982)

General Aspects of the Secondary Prevention of Myocardial Infarction

R. Rost

Institut für Kreislaufforschung und Sportmedizin, Köln, BRD

Introduction

Prior to talking of secondary prevention, this term must be closely defined. First it seems appropriate to distinguish between primary and secondary prevention. *Primary prevention* should be understood as the attempt to prevent coronary heart disease (CHD), whereas the term *secondary prevention* is used for measures that aim at stopping the progression of CHD, independent of the occurrence of myocardial infarction (MI).

The significance of risk factors may be different in primary and secondary prevention. A therapy which may be useful in primary prevention, can be useless after the clinical manifestation of the disease. On the other hand, there is no necessity to distinguish between primary, secondary and tertiary prevention, as is done by some authors who use different definitions [2, 8, 21, 26]as far as CHD is concerned.

However it is very difficult to make a sharp distinction between primary and secondary risk factors. We do not know whether the most widely accepted risk factors in CHD have the same significance in primary prevention compared with their role as prognostic factors after MI. There is some evidence that hypercholesterolemia, smoking habits and obesity may not have the same impact after MI. This may also be true of protective factors. The formation of collateral vessels through the influence of physical training probably does not play a role in healthy hearts, but may prove to be an important factor in CHD patients.

A distinction should also be made between rehabilitation and secondary prevention. Rehabilitation enables the patient to overcome the consequences of his disease, whereas secondary prevention should follow as the second phase to stop deterioration as effectively as possible.

The risk factors taken into consideration are modifiable (or questionably modifiable) and nonmodifiable ones. Factors which cannot be altered are those of age, sex, and genetic and ethnic origin. The group of modifiable factors are hypertension, hypercholesterolemia, diabetes and hyperuricemia, and external factors such as behavioral patterns, lifestyle, smoking habits, lack of exercise, diet, obesity and psychological factors. However, this classical conception of risk factors, which is also valid for primary prevention, has to be completed in the case of secondary prevention by additional factors which are caused by CHD or other cardiac diseases, such as cardiac enlargement, extension of myocardial damage, arrhythmias, myocardial failure, association with other vascular disorders (cerebral peripheral) and clinical symptoms such as unstable angina and others.

Taking into consideration the risk factors, the main objectives of secondary prevention can be divided into four groups:

(1) Interventions to change some behavioral patterns, such as: reasonable diet, antismoking program, physical training, control of body weight, avoidance or control of psychological stress.

(2) Medical treatment of internal risk factors, e.g. hypertension, hypercholesterolemia, diabetes, hyperuricemia.

(3) Medical treatment of cardiovascular disorders caused by CHD such as heart failure, arrhythmia, angina.

(4) Medical interventions on possible mechanisms of reinfarction or sudden death, such as anticoagulant therapy, platelet-suppressing therapy, coronary bypass surgery and aneurysmectomy.

Comprehensive Secondary Prevention

The most crucial points of comprehensive secondary prevention will be briefly discussed.

Diet and Weight Control

The general dietary recommendations for a patient after MI generally include a reduced intake of calories, fat, refined carbohydrates and an increased intake of animal proteins. The main goal is the control of body weight and metabolic disorders, such as diabetes and hypercholesterolemia. However, the scientific basis of these recommendations is not well established. Investigations have been carried out, predominantly into the connection between plasma lipid levels and MI. Whereas these investigations showed that decreased lipid levels are significant in primary prevention, they do not appear to exert an influence on the frequency of reinfarction. An association between cholesterol and reinfarction rate was found by *Jenkins* et al. [14] as well as by the Oslo heart study [19]. No influence was shown by *Elmfeldt* et al. [6], *Frank* [7], and others. But in spite of these results, there is sufficient evidence to make dietary recommendations, especially since they do not have any adverse effect on health.

Even as a method to control body weight, the use of a reasonable diet is questionable. As is generally known, obesity in itself cannot be considered as a risk factor in primary prevention, but it aggravates hypertension, hyperglycemia and hyperuricemia. The same is true in secondary prevention. *Norris* et al. [23] did not find any influence of obesity on mortality in a follow-up study after MI. However, in the case of secondary prevention, body weight control has to be recommended in patients with internal risk factors, such as hypertonia and hyperglycemia.

Antismoking Program

Whereas the increased risk of the smoker to suffer a MI is generally accepted, the discussion about the value of nonsmoking in secondary prevention has been open for many years. Some studies failed to emphasize the decreased risk of reinfarction in patients who stopped smoking after their first attack. Meanwhile, a number of studies are available which clearly show the value of stopping smoking. *Shapiro* et al [28] found a twice higher mortality in those patients who continued to smoke. Similar findings have been demonstrated more recently by the Goeteborg group. It has been stated by some authors that the association between smoking habits and reinfarction is only secondary to the personality pattern. However, the studies of *Jenkins* et al. [13, 14] and *Vedin* et al. [32] clearly show that the smokers risk does not depend on his personality. Therefore, the postinfarction patient should be urgently advised to stop smoking

Physical Activity

A definitive proof of the influence of physical training on CHD is still lacking. On the other hand, physical exercise is the accepted part of all rehabilitation programs. The reasons which have to be looked for are the psychological effects, the increase in performance capacity and the decrease of the sympathetic drive on the cardiovascular system.

Psychosocial Stress

The role of the psychological stress is one of the most controversial topics in primary as well as in secondary prevention. The question whether there is a pronounced MI personality or whether a first or second MI can be prevented using psychological techniques cannot be answered on the basis of current scientific data.

Medical Treatment

Intervention aimed at limiting infarct size and myocardial damage: even though the Goeteborg group demonstrated that primary risk factors such as hypertension, hyperlipidemia or smoking habits are more important for the long-term prognosis than the size of MI, the degree of myocardial damage has to be considered as an important risk factor. A number of clinical studies demonstrate that cardiac enlargement and cardiac failure in MI patients worsen the prognosis [29, 31]. Therefore, in our opinion, the standard therapy of digitalization and diuretics constitutes a very important part of secondary prevention along with modern sophisticated clinical techniques to diminish MI size. The same applies for the simple and complicated techniques for the early detection of heart failure.

Control of Arrhythmias

There is strong evidence that a high percentage of sudden deaths following MI is obviously due to 'malignant' uncontrolled arrhythmias [27]. There is also evidence that many forms of arrhythmias may aggravate the natural course of CHD after MI. Whereas some authors consider that arrhythmias impair the prognosis of post-MI patients, independent of the severity of CHD [20], others have demonstrated that the predictive influence of arrhythmias is related to the presence of other risk factors, such as cardiac failure, cardiomegaly, high blood pressure and others [5, 16, 25]. It has been shown that ventricular premature beats have a predictive value in post-MI patients, especially when they occur frequently or when they are complex [17, 22].

Despite these convincing data, the ongoing discussions on secondary prevention with antiarrhythmic drugs offer controversial and conflicting results. WHO studies on myocardial infarction and sudden death failed to provide consistent and conclusive data [36]. However, even though more clinical investigations on the effect of antiarrhythmic treatment seem to be necessary, it would be unreasonable to withhold the constant observation and treatment of arrhythmias in these patients.

Control of Hypertension

Whereas the importance of hypertension as a risk factor is unquestionable, there is no clear evidence for the time being that the treatment of hypertension will reduce the risk of MI in hypertensive patients. *Heyden* [12] presented two new studies demonstrating the value of antihypertensive treatment in primary prevention only recently.

The influence of hypertension and the effect of treatment in hypertensive post-MI patients are even more controversial. However, the change which could be observed in the assessment of antihypertensive treatment in primary prevention, as well as the fact that a number of trials demonstrate a higher reinfarction rate in hypertensive patients compared to normotensive ones [7, 9, 13], stress the necessity of antihypertensive treatment in hypertensive MI patients as an important part of secondary prevention.

Control of Metabolic Disorders

There is no doubt that treatment will be necessary in diabetic patients. However, the question still remains whether such a control really does prevent further atherosclerotic complications. Some authors described not only the effects of pharmacological treatment on the long-term prognosis of patients with diabetes mellitus, but also mentioned that some drugs, e.g. tolbutamides, have a possible secondary preventive effect after MI. However, the results are conflicting [24].

Also the treatment of hypothyroidism and hyperuricemia may have preventive value in some cases. About the effects of lipid-lowering drugs, the results are controversial and disappointing. There is no clear proof that the decrease in plasma lipid levels by those substances really has a positive influence on the prognosis of MI patients.

Anticoagulant Therapy

The numerous investigations into the effects of anticoagulant therapy failed to give evidence of an improved long-term prognosis of MI patients. Even if there are some positive studies, the use of anticoagulants has to be balanced against hemorrhagic complications [3, 9, 11].

A new approach to influence thrombopoesis is the administration of platelet – suppressing drugs. Whereas the results with dipyridamole seemed to be disappointing, acetylsalicylic acid seems – according to a number of studies – to prevent sudden death to some extent. Positive results were also obtained with sulfinpyrazine, however, these studies have to be confirmed by further trials [4, 6, 15].

Beta-Blocking Therapy

Among all pharmacological drugs which may be valid in secondary prevention, the beta-blockers certainly can be considered as the most important ones. There are a number of studies indicating a reduction of sudden death as well as of the frequency of reinfarction under chronic treatment by beta-blockers. The results may be based on the antiarrhythmic as well as on the oxygen-saving effect of beta-blockade [1, 10, 18, 33].

Coronary Surgery and Aneurysmectomy

Aorto-coronary bypass surgery becomes an increasingly accepted method in rehabilitation. The main clinical indication remains the relief of intractable pain. As far as the long-term prognosis is concerned, the results are still not clear. There are only certain forms of anatomic lesions in which decreased mortality could be observed. Uncontrolled studies also suggest that the mortality rate after MI can be reduced in those patients who undergo operations for cardiac conditions and lesions, such as post-MI ventricular aneurysms, post-MI ventricular septal defect or post-MI mitral valve incompetence [30, 35].

References

1 Balcon, R.; Jewitt, D. E.; Davies, J. P. F.; Oram, S.: A controlled trial of propranolol in acute myocardial infarction. Lancet, *ii:* 917 (1966).

2 Barker, D. J. P.: Practical epidemiology; 2nd ed. (Churchill, Livingstone, Edinburgh 1976).

3 Breddin, K.; Loew, D.; Lechner, K.; Oberla, K.; Walter, E.: Secondary prevention of myocardial infarction: comparison of acetylsalicylic acid, phenoprocoumon and placebo; in A multicenter two-year prospective study. 24th Annu. Meet. Committee of Thrombosis and Haemostasis, Leuwen 1979 (in press).

4 Craven, L. L.: Experiences with aspirin-acetylsalicylic acid in the non-specific prophylaxis of coronary thrombosis. Miss. Vall. med. J. *75:* 38 (1953).

5 Denborough, M. A.; Lovell, R. R. H.; Nestel, P. J.; Goble, A. J.: Arrhythmias and late sudden death after myocardial infarction. Lancet *i:* 386 (1968).

6 Elmfeldt, D.; Wilhelmsen, L.; Vedin, A.; Wilhelmsson, C.; Hjalmarson, A.; Bergstrand, R.; Sanne, H.: General aspects of secondary prevention after myocardial infarction. Cardiology *62:* 74 (1977).

7 Frank, Ch. W.: The course of coronary heart disease: factors related to prognosis. Bull. N. Y. Acad. Med. *44:* 900 (1968).

8 Garnham, J, C,; May, G. S.; Abu-Zeid, H.: Secondary prevention after myocardial infarction; in Gross, Modulation of sympathetic tone in the treatment of cardiovascular diseases (Huber, Bern 1979).

9 Gifford, R. H.; Feistein, A. P.: A critique of methodology in studies of anticoagulant therapy for acute myocardial infarction. New. Engl. J. Med. *280:* 351 (1969).

10 Grenn, K. G.: Reduction in mortality after myocardial infarction with long-term beta-adrenoreceptor blockade. Multicentre International Study. Supplementary report. Br. Med. J. 419 (1977).

11 Gross, H.; Vaid, A. K.; Levine, H. S.; Hasson, J.: Anticoagulant therapy in myocardial infarction. An overview of methodology. Am. J. Med. *52:* 421 (1972).

12 Heyden, S.: Präventive Kardiologie. Studienreihe Boehringer, Mannheim (1981).

13 Jenkins, C. D.; Zyzanski, S. J.; Rosenman, R. H.; Cleveland, G. B.: Association of coronary-prone behaviour scores with recurrence of coronary heart disease. J. chron. Dis. *24:* 601 (1971).

14 Jenkins, C. D.; Zyzanski, S. J.; Rosenman, J. M.: Risk of new myocardial infarction in middel-aged men with manifest coronary heart disease. Circulation *53:* 342–347 (1976).

15 Kaegi, A.; Pineo, J. F.; Shimiza, A.; Trivedi, H.; Hirsh, J.; Gent, M.: Arterio-venous shunt, thrombosis: prevention by sulphinpyrazone. New Engl. J. Med. *290:* 304 (1974).

16 Kitchin, A. H.; Pocock, S. J.: Prognosis of patients with acute myocardial infarction admitted to a coronary care unit. II. Survival after hospital discharge. Br. Heart J. *39:* 1167 (1977).

17 Kotler, M. N.; Tabatznick, B.; Mower, M. N.; Tominaga, S.: Prognostic significance of ventricular ectopic beats with respect to sudden death in the late postinfarction period. Circulation *47:* 959 (1973).

18 Lambert, D. M. D.: Long-term survival on beta-receptor-blocking drugs in general practice. A three-year prospective study; in Birdwood, Burley, Hypertension – its nature and treatment. An international symposium, p. 283 (Ciba Laboratories, Horsham 1975).

19 Leren, P.: The Oslo diet-heart study: 11 year-report. Circulation *42:* 935–942 (1970).

20 Locksley, R.; Moss, A. H.; DeCamilla, J.; Mietlowsky, W.: Prognostic grading and significance of VPBs after myocardial infarction. Circulation *50:* suppl. 3, p. 121 (1974).

21 McMahon, B,; Pugh, T. F.: Epidemiology: principles and methods (Little, Brown, Boston 1970).

22 Moss, A. J.; DeCamilla, J.; Engstrom, F.; Hoffmann, W.; Odoroff, C.; Davis, H.: The posthospital phase of myocardial infarction. Identification of patients with increased mortality risk. Circulation *49:* 460 (1974).

23 Norris, R. M.; Cauchery, D. E.; Mercer, C. J.; Scott, P. J.: Prognosis after myocardial infarction. Six-year follow-up. Br. Heart J. *36:* 786 (1974).

24 Paasikivi, J.: Long-term tolbutamide treatment after myocardial infarction. Acta med. scand., suppl. 507 (1970).

25 Pell, S.; D'Alonzo: Immediate mortality and five years' survival of employed men with first myocardial infarction. New. Engl. J. Med. *270:* 915 (1964).

26 Pflanz, M.: Epidemiologie und Präventivmedizin. Dt. Ärztebl. *68:* 467 (1971).

27 Schwartz, P. J.; Wolf, S.: QT interval prolongation as predictor of sudden death in patients with myocardial infarction. Circulation *57:* 1074 (1978).

28 Shapiro, S.; Weinblatt, E.; Frank, C.: The HIP study of incidence and prognosis of coronary heart disease. The Health Insurance Plan of Greater New York (New York 1970).
29 Shell, W. E.; Sobel, B. E.: Infarct size index: an effective indicator of prognosis after myocardial infarction. Circulation *48:* suppl. IV, p. 39 (1973).
30 Shore, T. R.; Johnson, D. W.: Indications for coronary artery surgery and patient selection; in Chung, Controversy in cardiology, p. 152 (Springer, New York 1976).
31 Sobel, B. E.; Bresnahan, G. F.; Shell, W. E.; Yoder, R. D.: Estimation of infarct size in man and its relation to prognosis. Circulation *46:* 640 (1972).
32 Vedin, A.; Wilhelmsson, C.; Elmfeldt, D.; Save-Soderberg, J.; Tibblin, G.; Wilhelmsen, L.: Deaths and non-fatal reinfarctions during two years' follow-up after myocardial infarction. Acta med. scand. *198:* 353 (1975).
33 Wilhelmsson, C.; Vedin, J. A.; Wilhelmsen, L.; Tibblin, G.; Werko, L.: Reduction of sudden deaths after myocardial infarction by treatment with alprenolol. Lancet *ii:* 1157 (1974).
34 Wilhelmsson, C.; Vedin, J. A.; Wilhelmsen, L.; Tibblin, G.; Werko, L.; Wedel, H.: Deaths and non-fatal reinfarctions during two year follow-up. Acta med. scand., suppl. 575, p. 19 (1975).
35 World Health Organization: The long-term effects of coronary bypass surgery. Report on a working group, The Hague 1977 (WHO Regional Office for Europe, Copenhagen 1979).
36 World Health Organization: Coronary care in the community. Report on a working group, Torremolinos 1976 (WHO Regional Office for Europe, Copenhagen 1976).

Prof. Dr. R. Rost, Institut für Kreislaufforschung und Sportmedizin,
Carl-Diem-Weg, D–5000 Köln 41 (FRG)

Adv. Cardiol., vol. 31, pp. 120–128 (Karger, Basel 1982)

Rehabilitation Programmes as Secondary Prevention: A Community Approach

Veikko Kallio

Rehabilitation Research Centre of the Social Insurance Institution, Turku, Finland

Rehabilitation as defined by a recent WHO Expert Committee on Disability Prevention and Rehabilitation [4] includes all measures aimed at reducing the impact of disabling and handicapping conditions, and at enabling the disabled and handicapped to achieve social integration. The disabled and handicapped themselves, their families, and the communities they live in, should be involved in the planning and implementation of services related to rehabilitation. Social integration is viewed as the active participation of disabled and handicapped persons in the mainstream of community life.

Community-based rehabilitation was defined by the Expert Committee to involve measures taken at the community level to use and build on the resources of the community. These resources include the impaired, disabled, and handicapped persons themselves, their families, and their community as a whole.

Whereas social integration is thus considered to be the main aim of rehabilitation, it is important to emphasize that as regards chronic diseases, such as advanced forms of coronary heart disease, secondary preventive measures, if available, should be incorporated into the rehabilitation programme. While the aim of rehabilitation, i.e. the social integration of the patient, will usually be achieved within a year after an acute myocardial infarction (MI) and often after a relatively short programme of active rehabilitation, the secondary preventive programmes may have to be continued much longer.

According to the Joint Recommendations by the ISFC Scientific Councils on Arteriosclerosis, Epidemiology and Prevention, and Rehabilitation, survivors of MI too often receive inadequate follow-up after

Table I. Cumulative 2-year mortality and non-fatal reinfarctions after MI in the intervention and reference groups [20]

	Intervention (n = 96), %	Reference (n = 85), %	p
Non-fatal reinfarction	11	26	<0.025
Coronary deaths	9	15	NS
All deaths	13	16	NS
New coronary events	21	41	<0.05

recovery. 'We believe that planned and sustained care can substantially improve their rehabilitation and prognosis' [19]. This statement about prognosis is substantiated by the results of the Gothenburg group which showed that organized care at a Post-Infarction Clinic, even without a formal rehabilitation programme, may bring about a reduction of recurrences [20] (table I).

Rehabilitation programmes have often been primarily concerned with physical activation and training of the patient. The results of early activation and physical exercise programmes after an MI have been encouraging, although controlled studies have shown that life expectancy is not prolonged [2, 7, 10, 13]. During recent years increased emphasis has been put on other aspects of life-style as well, such as health education aimed at having patients stop smoking, lose weight if indicated, change their diet to reduce fat intake, and reduce stress and anxiety in their lives. To reach all patients at a cost that society can afford, a community approach is necessary. Several programmes currently in progress make use of community resources, sometimes in cooperation with specialized rehabilitation institutes [6, 14, 15, 18, 22]. The Hamburg model, developed by *Krasemann* [14], provides an example of how to organize a programme for selected patients based on cooperation among hospitals, Rehabilitation Clinics, primary physicians, and sports clubs. The results are reported to be positive, although effects of secondary prevention have not been shown (table II).

In general, development of a community programme requires careful planning and organization [1, 15, 22]. The programme should make use of existing health services and should be integrated into the system of health services already available [21]. To insure that every patient will be included in the programme there must be continuity from hospital to community

Table II. Effects of organized group rehabilitation with special emphasis on physical exercise [14]

Risk factors	++
Physical working capacity	++
Quality of life	+++
Adaptation to work	++
Reinfarctions	(+)
Longevity	?

services. Proper emphasis should be given to the education and training of health-related personnel in rehabilitation and in communication skills. The patient's family should be appropriately involved.

Some experiences from Finland might be helpful in illustrating how a country-wide community-based programme has been built up, step by step, during the last few years.

During the early 1970s data on the incidence of acute MI were collected through community Ischaemic Heart Disease registers according to a protocol developed by the WHO. These data confirmed the findings of earlier studies showing incidence figures that were the highest in Europe [16]. These incidence figures varied considerably among the centres [17], with the incidence of new cases of MI being highest in the eastern part of Finland, in North Karelia (fig. 1).

This awareness of the high incidence of coronary heart disease, particularly in North Karelia, gave the impetus for launching the North Karelia Project [3]. The project was to consist of a systematic comprehensive community programme aimed at getting cardiovascular diseases under control in the county of North Karelia, a mainly rural area with some 180,000 inhabitants. This programme was also to include rehabilitation and secondary prevention. An attempt was made to direct and develop existing health services to meet the needs of the programme [18]. The programme consisted of systematic long-term medical follow-up at the outpatient MI clinic of a hospital and of decentralized local group rehabilitation with special emphasis on secondary prevention. The main components of the programme were patient education and submaximal physical exercise aimed at reducing known secondary risk factors and at the improvement of general well-being. During the 5-year programme period the incidence of recurrent infarctions dropped by 25%. The trend in the 1-year total mortality rate among patients with a recurrent infarction also declined (fig. 2).

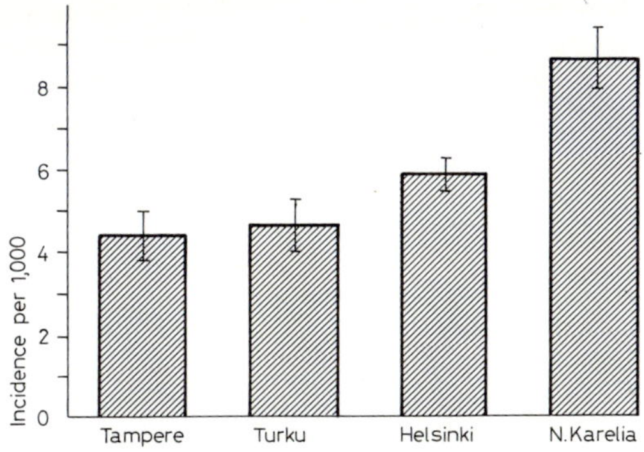

Fig. 1. Incidence of AMI (verified and possible) in four Finnish Ischaemic Heart Disease register areas in 1973 [17].

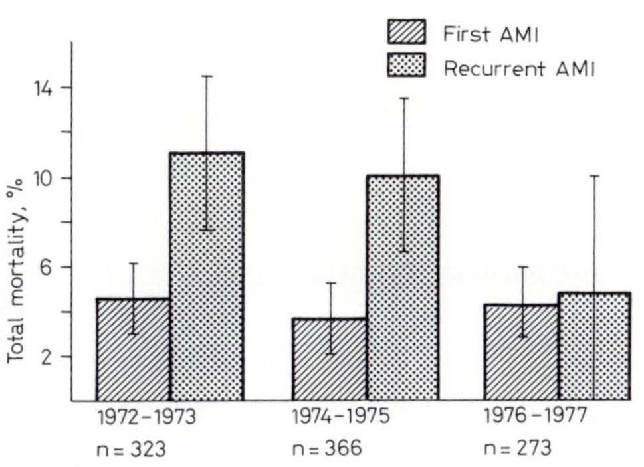

Fig. 2. Changes in 1-year total mortality (%) during 1972–1977 among male MI patients (North Karelia Project) [18].

Launched almost concomitantly with the North Karelia Project was a project, coordinated by the WHO, that studied the effects of comprehensive rehabilitation and secondary prevention in patients who had had an MI [5]. The Finnish study was carried out in two centres, one in Turku and the other in Helsinki [12]. The aim of the study was to compare the impact of comprehensive up-to-date intervention after an MI with the impact of services provided after an MI by the existing health care system. The Finnish series consisted of 375 consecutive patients younger than 65 years who had survived a verified AMI diagnosed according to WHO criteria [8]. At dismissal from hospital the patients were randomly allocated to an intervention or to a control group. The groups were comparable in age, and

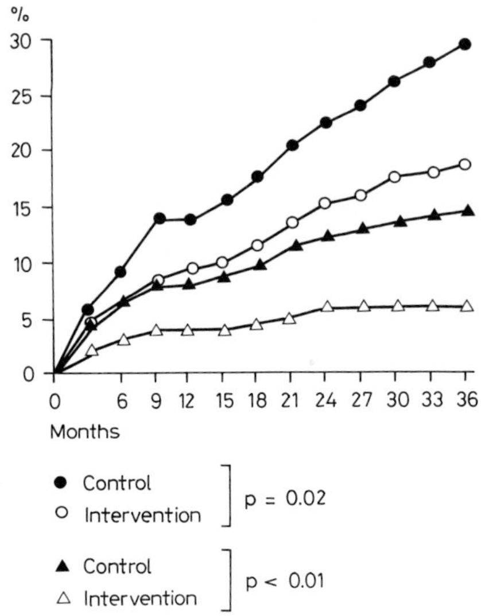

Fig. 3. Cumulative coronary mortality (●, ○) and sudden deaths (▲,△) during 3 years after MI in the intervention and control groups [12].

in the distribution of various prognostic variables and characteristics at discharge from hospital.

While in hospital all patients were given general advice and information on rehabilitation and on secondary preventive measures. The 1-year rehabilitation programme for the intervention group started about 2 weeks after discharge from hospital, i.e. about 4 weeks after the acute event.

The patients in the control group were treated on their own initiave by their own doctors, and were seen by the study team only once a year during the 3-year follow-up period. Only a few of them participated in any organized rehabilitation programme.

At the end of the first year follow-up, there were significant differences between the groups, the intervention group having lower mean values in body weight, serum cholesterol, serum triglycerides, and systolic and diastolic blood pressure. Most of these differences were still present 3 years after the AMI. At the same time, coronary mortality declined significantly in the intervention group due mainly to the decrease in mortality from sudden death, as seen in figure 3. According to preliminary results, this trend still persisted at 6 years follow-up. Patients with a relatively good prognosis after the MI seemed to benefit most from the programme. The

Table III. Cumulative 3-year coronary mortality after MI in different age groups in the intervention (I) and control (C) groups [12]

Age groups, years	Number		Coronary mortality, %	
	I	C	I	C
<49	40	54	2.5	25.9**
50–54	42	36	23.8	25.0
55–59	47	42	23.4	31.0
60–64	48	54	20.8	35.2

**p<0.01.

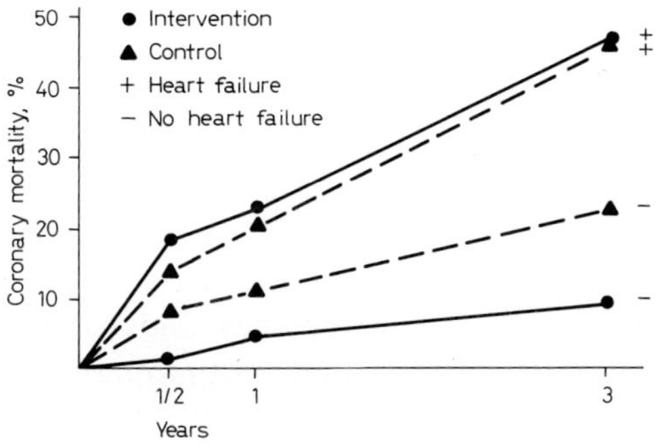

Fig. 4. Cardiac failure recorded in hospital and subsequent 3-year coronary mortality after MI in the intervention and control groups [12].

difference in coronary (and total) death rates between the intervention and control groups was greatest in patients younger than 50 years (table III). On the other hand, cardiac failure recorded during the hospital stay carried an equally serious prognosis in both the intervention and control groups (fig. 4).

Since the study had shown that the intervention programme was effective in secondary prevention as well as for improved social integration of the patient, the basic elements of the intervention programme, that is, organized after-care, optimum medical control, health education and an advised or supervised programme of physical exercise, were chosen to be tested on the community level. A new controlled trial was launched to study the feasibility and the effects of such a community programme when carried out by the outpatient services of the five participating hospitals and by

Table IV. Cumulative 1-year mortality and non-fatal reinfarctions after MI in the community-based and institute-based rehabilitation groups [11]

	Community (n = 228), %	Institute (n = 228), %
Non-fatal reinfarction	6.0	4.5
Coronary mortality	8.8	8.3
Total mortality	9.2	9.2
New coronary events	14.8	12.8

community-based voluntary organizations, such as the local Heart Associations [11]. The effectiveness of the community programme was compared with that of a 2-week residential rehabilitation programme and out-patient services provided by a specialized rehabilitation centre. Altogether 456 consecutive patients with first MI below the age of 65 were involved in the study, 228 in each group. The community approach turned out to be feasible. Preliminary results indicate that the cumulative total and coronary mortality 1 year after the MI was about the same in both groups and almost the same as in the intervention group in our previous study (table IV). Conclusions at this stage of the study must be drawn with caution. It does appear, however, that as far as short-term survival and morbidity are concerned, the effects of an organized, community-based and relatively simple programme during the first 3 months after an MI compare well with those achieved with a more sophisticated programme provided by a special institute.

At the same time as these research results became available, a country-wide implementation of rehabilitation and secondary prevention measures was started, financed through a nation-wide fund-raising campaign, Operation Red Heart, that was organized by the Lions International in Finland. The programme provides hospital health education, outpatient follow-up by the treating hospital during the first 6 months after discharge, and guidance group activities, including physical exercise sessions organized by the local community. Attempts were made to integrate these activities into the existing system of health services so that they would become a part of the routine services. Experiences gained so far have been encouraging. Evaluation studies of this country-wide effort are under way [9].

It can be concluded that rehabilitation programmes, as carried out now in many countries, have given promising results as regards social integration and quality of life after an MI. Measures aimed at secondary prevention and incorporated into the rehabilitation programmes constitute an important contribution toward promoting a healthy life-style. As recent studies suggest, these measures may well prove effective in reducing mortality or morbidity, or both, after an MI. Efforts along these lines should be continued.

A community approach, based on existing local health services and on other resources available in the community, is feasible and should be developed further in accordance with local needs and facilities.

References

1 Acker, J. E.: Medical benefits and concerns in cardiac rehabilitation; in Pollock, Schmidt, Heart disease and rehabilitation, pp. 654–662 (Houghton Mifflin, Boston 1979).

2 Bruce, R. A.: Progress in exercise cardiology; in Yu, Goodwin, Progress in cardiology; 3th ed., pp. 113–172 (Lea & Febiger, Philadelphia 1974).

3 World Health Organization: Community control of cardiovascular diseases, Evaluation of a comprehensive community programme for control of cardiovascular diseases in North Karelia, Finland 1972–1977 (National Public Health Laboratory of Finland & WHO, Copenhagen 1981).

4 World Health Organization: Disability prevention and rehabilitation. Report of the WHO Expert Committee on Disability Prevention and Rehabilitation. Tech. Rep. Ser. No. 668 (WHO, Geneva 1981).

5 World Health Organization: Evaluation of comprehensive rehabilitative and preventive programmes for patients after acute myocardial infarction. Report on two Working Groups, Prague 1971 and Moscow 1972 (WHO, Copenhagen 1973).

6 Halhuber, C.: Rehabilitation in ambulanten Koronargruppen. Ein human-ökologischer Ansatz; Rehabilitation und Prävention, vol. 13 (Springer, Berlin 1980).

7 Hellerstein, H. K.: Cardiac rehabilitation: a retrospective view; in Pollock, Schmidt, Heart disease and rehabilitation, pp. 509–520 (Houghton Mifflin, Boston 1979).

8 World Health Organization: Ischaemic heart disease registers. Report of the Fifth Working Group (WHO, Copenhagen 1971).

9 Järvinen, T.; Keskilä, T.; Luurila, O. J.: Operation Red Heart; in Järvinen, Keskilä, Luurila, Operaatio Punainen Sydän, pp. 133–138 (Operaatio Punainen Sydän-rahasto, Espoo 1981).

10 Kallio, V.: Results of rehabilitation in coronary patients; in König, Denolin, Cardiac rehabilitation, pp. 153–163 (Karger, Basel 1978).

11 Kallio, V.; Hämäläinen, H.; Vuori, I.; Arstila, M.; Aalto-Setälä, J.; Härmälä, V.; Kaarsalo, E.; Laurila, J.; Pere, E.; Leino, T.: Community approach in rehabilitation and secondary prevention after myocardial infarction; Publication of the Social Insurance Institution of Finland Series ML (with English summary) (in press, 1982).

12 Kallio, V.; Hämäläinen, H.; Hakkila, J.; Luurila, O. J.: Reduction in sudden deaths by a multifactorial intervention programme after acute myocardial infarction. Lancet *ii:* 1091–1094 (1979).

13 Kellermann, J. J.; Denolin, H.: Critical evaluation of cardiac rehabilitation. Proc. Scient. Meet. of Critical Evaluation of Cardiac Rehabilitation, Tel Aviv 1975. Biblthca cardiol., vol. 36 (Karger, Basel 1976).

14 Krasemann, E. O.: Die organisierte Herzinfarkt-Rehabilitation. Fortschr. Med. *97:* 1987–1990 (1979).

15 Miller, H. S.; Ribisl, P. M.; Adams, G. E.; Boone, W. T.: Community programs of cardiac rehabilitation; in Pollock, Schmidt, Heart disease and rehabilitation, pp. 480–495 (Houghton Mifflin, Boston 1979).

16 World Health Organization: Myocardial infarction community registers. Results of a WHO International collaborative study coordinated by the Regional Office for Europe (WHO, Copenhagen 1976).

17 Pohjola, S.; Siltanen, P.; Romo, M.; Haapakoski, J.; Salonen, J.; Puska, P.; Mustaniemi, H.; Ruosteenoja, R.; Arstila, M.; Kallio, V.: Sydäninfarktin esiintyvyys ja ennuste Suomessa vuonna 1973. Duodecim *96:* 18–31 (1980).

18 Salonen, J. T.; Puska, P.: A community programme for rehabilitation and secondary prevention for patients with acute myocardial infarction as part of a comprehensive community programme for control of cardiovascular diseases (North Karelia Project). Scand. J. Rehabil. Med. *12:* 33–42 (1980).

19 Secondary prevention in myocardial infarction survivors. Heart Beat *3:* 1–3 (1980).

20 Vedin, A.; Wilhelmsson, C.; Tibblin, G.; Wilhelmsen, L.: The postinfarction clinic in Göteborg, Sweden. Acta med. scand. *200:* 453–456 (1976).

21 Wenger, N. K.: The future of rehabilitation: a component of routine cardiac care; in König, Denolin, Cardiac rehabilitation, pp. 197–201 (Karger, Basel 1978).

22 Whitney, L. A.: Community dynamics of prevention and rehabilitation programs; in Long, Prevention and rehabilitation in ischemic heart disease, pp. 345–366 (Williams & Wilkins, Baltimore 1980).

Prof. V. Kallio, MD, Director, The Rehabilitation Research Centre of the Social Insurance Institution, Peltolantie 3, SF-20720 Turku 72 (Finland)

Adv. Cardiol., vol. 31, pp. 129–133 (Karger, Basel 1982)

Comparison of Methods for Determining Exercise Training Intensity for Cardiac Patients and Healthy Adults

M. L. Pollock, C. Foster, J. L. Rod, G. Wible

Cardiac Rehabilitation Program, Cardiovascular Disease Section, Department of Medicine, University of Wisconsin Medical School, Mount Sinai Medical Center, Milwaukee, Wisc., USA

Introduction

Several factors must be considered in an exercise prescription designed to improve cardiovascular fitness in either healthy individuals or cardiac patients. These include the frequency, duration, intensity and mode of the aerobic exercise [1, 2]. The most difficult factor to prescribe and to monitor is the intensity of exercise, primarily because direct measurement of relative oxygen uptake (VO_2) during exercise is impractical. The heart rate (HR) during exercise is often used as an index of exercise intensity. Two methods for prescribing exercise intensity on the basis of heart rate are in general use [2]. Method I represents the percent of the maximal HR attained calculated from 0 to peak HR (% max HR). Method II represents the percent difference between resting and maximal HR added to the resting HR as described by *Karvonen* et al. [3] (% max HR reserve). Although both techniques are used extensively, Method I yields a 10 to 30 beat/minute lower training HR value when calculated between 60 and 85 % of maximal HR [2]. The rating of perceived exertion (RPE) as described by *Borg* [4] has been used in graded exercise testing (GXT) and has been shown to be highly related to physiological variables such as blood lactate, pulmonary ventilation, HR, and VO_2. More recently, RPE has been used as an adjunct to HR in determining and monitoring exercise training [5, 6]. In using RPE for exercise prescription, values ranging from 12–13 (somewhat hard) to 15–16 (hard) have been suggested as a desireable training intensity to elicit an adequate training effect. The purpose of the present investigation was to compare the two HR methods for prescribing exercise, particularly as they are related to RPE.

Table I. Physical characteristics of the subjects

Group	n	Age, years	Height, cm	Weight, kg
Young healthy	51	28 ± 5	170 ± 11	71 ± 14
		(19–39)	(147–188)	(46–103)
Older healthy	42	54 ± 8	175 ± 11	81 ± 15
		(40–70)	(152–193)	(51–123)
Cardiac patients[1]	48	54 ± 10	174 ± 9	73 ± 11
		(35–73)	(154–194)	(46–98)

Data represent mean ± standard deviation (range in parentheses).
[1]Studied at hospital discharge, 12 ± 24 days postsurgery.

Material and Methods

48 patients with documented coronary artery disease and 93 healthy individuals were studied during symptom-limited GXT. Some characteristics of the subjects are provided in table I. All of the cardiac patients had undergone coronary artery bypass graft surgery and were studied at the time of hospital discharge 12 ± 4 days postoperatively.

GXT was performed on a treadmill using a modified (2-min stages) Naughton protocol [7]. The electrocardiogram (ECG) was monitored continuously and HR was measured from 12-lead ECG records obtained during the last 15 s of each minute of exercise. Blood pressure (BP) was measured by auscultation during the last 30 s of each exercise stage. RPE was measured using the Borg scale [4] during the last 5 s of each minute of exercise. Exercise was continued to symptoms (fatigue, dyspnea, 2^+ angina, claudication) or signs (3 mm ST depression over rest, inappropriate BP response, significant ectopic activity) of exertional intolerance.

Training HRs were calculated at 60, 70, and 85% of maximal HR (method I: 0 to peak) and % of maximal HR reserve (method II) for each group of subjects. Patients on beta-blocking medication were included in the series since we have previously [8] demonstrated that beta blockade does not influence the HR-RPE relationship. 25% of the patients were taking propranolol.

Results

Maximal GXT test results are presented in table II. The young healthy, older healthy and cardiac patients attained 94, 93 and 71% of their age predicted maximal HR, respectively. For coronary patients not on propranolol 74% of the age predicted maximal HR was attained. RPE at maximal exertion corresponded to a rating of very hard [17] to very, very

Table II. Results of the maximal treadmill test

	Heart rate (beats/min)		METs	RPE
	rest [1]	max.		
Young healthy	70 ± 14	181 ± 20	13 ± 2	19 ± 1
Older healthy	80 ± 15	150 ± 24	7 ± 3	18 ± 1
Cardiac patients	87 ± 13	118 ± 17	4 ± 1	17 ± 2

Data represent mean ± standard deviation.
[1] Data represent standing values.

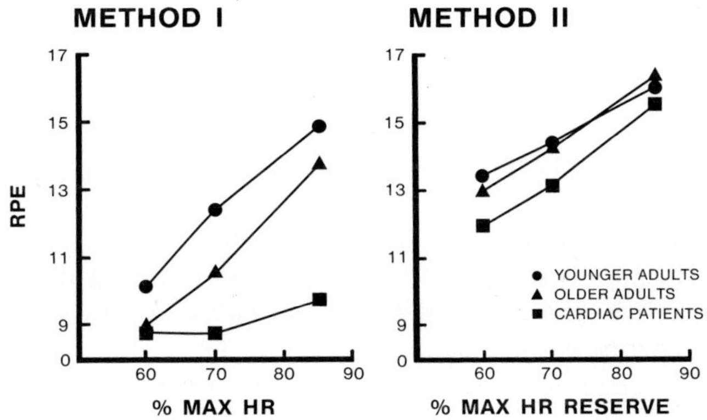

Fig. 1. Relationship between heart rate (HR) and perceived exertion (RPE) using two methods of calculating training heart rate. Percent max HR (method I) was calculated on the basis of the percentage of the difference between 0 and the peak HR attained. Percent max HR reserve (method II) was calculated according to *Karvonen* et al. [3] and represents the percent difference between the resting and maximal HR added to the resting HR.

hard [19]. This is consistent with fatigue as the predominant reason for test termination in approximately 90% of cases, including patients.

The relationship between training HR calculated by the two methods is presented in figure 1. Method I resulted in a significantly different percent of HR to RPE relationship for of each of the groups. This difference was most pronounced with the coronary patients. Also, compared to method II, the RPE at any given % HR was significantly lower. Method II resulted in a relatively consistent percent of HR-RPE relationship among all groups.

RPE averages ranged from 12–13 at 60% of max HR reserve to 15–16 at 85% of the max HR reserve.

Discussion

Training HRs are usually prescribed between 60 and 85% of either the % max HR (method I) or of the % max HR reserve (method II). These methods have been shown to be of utilitarian value when a direct HR-VO_2 relationship cannot be established [9]. *Davis and Convertino* [10] have demonstrated that method II is more accurate than method I in terms of yielding numerically equivalent values for relative VO_2 in young healthy students. Nonpublished data by *Kaufmann and Kasch* have shown the same relationship with middle-aged men. The RPE data from the present study, using three distinctly different populations, suggest that method II also produces more consistent results in a variety of populations.

If RPE values of 12–16 represent a desirable training range for both healthy adults and cardiac patients, then the consistency of the HR-RPE relationship among the groups using method II suggests validity of this technique compared to method I. Method I produces consistently lower values for RPE at any given percentage of the maximal HR. This was particularly true for the cardiac patients, and may be related to the low maximal HRs at this stage of recovery. Our experience with patients within 2 weeks of an acute clinical episode indicates that inpatients rate early ambulation between 11 and 12 on the RPE scale [11]. Outpatients within the first 3 months following hospital discharge rate aerobic training activities from 12–13 [5]. It is of interest that despite the patients resting tachycardia, low HR and consequently small HR reserve, method II yielded essentially the same relationship with RPE as noted in the healthy subjects with their much greater HR reserve. Whether this relationship extends to the relative VO_2 as with young normals [10] remains to be determined.

In summary the results of the present investigation suggest that the % max HR reserve method of *Karvonen* et al. [3] for prescribing exercise training HR is well related to the range of RPE which is usually recommended for training. This relationship is consistent across a variety of populations suggesting that this method of calculating training HR is inherently superior to the 0 to peak method. The data suggest that percent max HR calculated by the 0 to peak method may be too conservative for use with both cardiac patients and healthy adults.

References

1 American College of Sports Medicine: Position stand on the recommended quantity and quality of exercise for developing and maintaining fitness in healthy adults. Med. Sci. Sports *10:* vii-x (1978).

2 Pollock, M. L.; Ward, A.; Foster, C.: Heart disease and rehabilitation, pp. 413–445 (Wiley, New York 1979).

3 Karvonen, M.; Kentala, K.; Mustala, O.: The effects of training on heart rate: a longitudinal study. Annls Med. exp. Biol. Fenn. *35:* 307–315 (1957).

4 Borg, G. A.: Perceived exertion. A note on history and methods. Med. Sci. Sports *5:* 90–93 (1973).

5 Gutmann, M. C.; Squires, R. W.; Pollock, M. L.; Foster, C.; Anholm, J.: Perceived exertion-heart rate relationship during exercise testing and training in cardiac patients. J. card. Rehab. *1:* 52–95 (1981).

6 Smutok, M. A.; Skrinar, G. S.; Pandolf, K. B.: Exercise intensity: Subjective regulation by perceived exertion. Archs phys. Med. Rehabil. *61:* 569–574 (1980).

7 Patterson, J. A.; Naughton, J.; Pietras, R. J.; Gunnar, R. M.: Treadmill exercise in assessment of the functional capacity of patients with cardiac disease. Am. J. Cardiol. *30:* 757–762 (1972).

8 Squires, R. W.; Rod, J. L.; Pollock, M. L.; Foster, C.; Schmidt, D. H.: Effect of propranolol on perceived exertion during graded exercise testing soon after myocardial revascularization surgery. Med. Sci. Sports Ex. (in press).

9 Wilmore, J. H.; Haskell, W.: Use of the heart rate-energy expenditure relationship in the individual prescription of exercise. Am. J. clin. Nutr. *24:* 1186–1192 (1971).

10 Davis, J. A.; Convertino, V. A.: A comparison of heart rate methods for predicting endurance training intensity. Med. Sci. Sports *7:* 295–298 (1975).

11 Faraher, W.; Grevenow, P.; Pollock, M. L.; Squires, R. W.; Foster, C.; Johnson, W. D.; Schmidt, D. H.: Medical problems and physiologic responses during supervised inpatient cardiac rehabilitation. The coronary artery bypass graft surgery patient. Heart Lung *11:* 248–255 (1982).

M. L. Pollock, PhD, Director, Cardiac Rehabilitation Department and Human Performance Laboratory, Mount Sinai Medical Center, 950 North Twelfth Street, Milwaukee, WI 53233 (USA)

Adv. Cardiol., vol. 31, pp. 134–137 (Karger, Basel 1982)

Cardiac Rehabilitation as a Secondary Preventive Measure – Endpoints

The Logic of Desirability and Availability

Jan J. Kellermann

Cardiac Evaluation and Rehabilitation Institute, Chaim Sheba Medical Center, Tel Hashomer, Israel

In order to assess the efficacy of a therapeutic modality, well-designed randomized trials are necessary. There is no controversy as to scientific requirements needed to prove that a certain therapy or management has a measurable effect. If the goal of such a trial is 'hard endpoints' (i. e. disease or death), it is necessary to conduct such studies for a long period of time with a large sample size, in order to achieve meaningful results. The implication of comprehensive rehabilitation programs in patients with coronary heart disease remains still controversial as to prevention of mortality and morbidity [1, 2].

For the past decade many scientists, cardiologists, national and international institutions stressed the urgent need of a well-controlled, randomized trial, in order to find an answer to this latter question [8, 9]. Despite the evidence that such trials are very expensive and their cost-benefit effectiveness has yet to be established, nobody was prepared to compromise with a more flexible and less rigid scientific approach.

Requirements – Problems – Biases

The following aspects must be taken into consideration [11]:

(a) It is desirable to conduct a randomized trial taking into consideration all the aspects of a pure scientific procedure. In order to perform such a trial we have to face a number of very difficult problems, such as *exact dosage, patients compliance* and *contaminations.* Furthermore, endpoints must be clearly defined because there may be a number of detection biases, identification difficulties and a lack of unity for the classification of symptoms and signs.

(b) The other problems consist of the so-called preintervention baseline state. When dealing with a multifactorial disease such as coronary heart disease, one must be especially aware to assess constantly not only the severity of symptoms and the symptoms combination, but also the rate of progress. As a consequence of cointerventions, changes in the titration of dosage may be necessary.

(c) In coronary heart disease with a pathogenesis of atherosclerosis of coronary vessels, a great number of risk factors may influence the natural course of the disease [3]. The problem of 'the therapeutic baseline state' may present an obstacle almost impossible to overcome. The following risk factors may eventually influence prognosis, either by interaction or by sudden uncontrollable events [2]: heredity, impaired lipid metabolism, diabetes, hypertension, smoking habits, obesity, physical inactivity, personality traits and behavior patterns, psychosocial stresses, ethnic-cultural backgrounds.

Comprehensive Rehabilitation

Comprehensive rehabilitation programs [3, 6] based on risk factor modification, exercise training, drug intervention, counselling and especially on a close follow-up enabling a constant assessment of clinical variables by means of noninvasive and eventualy invasive methods, have proved the following:

Exercise Therapy [5, 7, 10]: Physical work capacity and stroke volume is enhanced as a consequence of an effective physical training program. The HR and the double product decreases for a given work-load. The maximal oxygen uptake increases. In about 20% of patients with angina pectoris the angina threshold heart rate and ejection fraction increases, especially after intensive training.

Psychological Effects [4, 12]: Anxiety and fear decreases, Self-confidence increases. A more balanced emotional stability is achieved. The socioeconomic status improves. The emotional response to sudden unexpected psychological stresses is lessened.

Close follow-up involving at least twice yearly clinical reassessments and urgent appliance of diagnostic procedures whenever requested, enables improved management, better timing and initiation of therapy.

The use of antihypertensive, antiarrhythmic, antianginal and antidiabetic drugs, if indicated together with the modification of risk factors, contributes to a more efficient intervention.

All these undertakings, which are part of a supervised comprehensive rehabilitation program, may cause difficult problems of cointerventions in the individual patient. This approach may influence directly outcome events, either as a consequence of a single therapeutic procedure, or as a result of comprehensive therapy. Prognosis may therefore be influenced in all these patients who are reacting beneficially to therapy and who are eventually preselected due to a consequent adherence to longtime programs of this kind.

It is mandatory that any results of randomized studies can be taken into consideration only when their duration extends to a large number of years. In most of the randomized studies undertaken to date, the ambitions to achieve final hard endpoint criterions, proved to be a 'mission impossible'. What we have to accept is the fact that a great number of biases cannot be eliminated when intervening in different groups of patients with CHD. We should stop fighting Don Quixote wars and adapt ourselves to what is achievable. We should pay more attention to so-called 'soft' endpoints, such as quality of survival and not survival itself. Whether or not it is possible to scientifically measure 'soft' endpoints remains at this stage to be demonstrated.

References

1 Kellermann, J. J.; Denolin, H.: Critical evaluation of cardiac rehabilitation. Biblthca Cardiol., vol. 36 (Karger, Basel 1977).

2 Kellermann, J. J.: Can we improve the prognosis of coronary heart disease; in Mathes, Halhuber, Current problems in cardiac rehabilitation, pp. 123–129 (Springer, Berlin 1982).

3 Kellermann, J. J.: Rehabilitation of patients with coronary heart disease. Prog. cardiovasc. Dis. *17:* 303–328 (1975).

4 Wintner, I.; Kellermann, J. J.: Psychological factors in cardiac rehabilitation; in Stocksmeier, Psychological approach to the rehabilitation of coronary patients, pp. 156–172 (Springer, Berlin 1976).

5 Kellermann, J. J.; Ben-Ari, E.; Chayet, M.; Lapidot, C.; Drory, Y.; Fisman, E.: Cardiocirculatory response to different types of training in patients with angina pectoris. Cardiology *62:* 218–231 (1977).

6 Kellermann, J. J.: Cardiac rehabilitation: reminiscences, international variations, experiences. J. card. Rehabil. *1:* 43–50 (1981).

7 Clausen, J. P.: Circulatory adjustments to dynamic exercise and effect of physical training in normal subjects and in patients with coronary artery disease; in Sonnenblick, Lesch, Exercise and heart disease, pp. 39–75 (Grune & Stratton, New York 1977).
8 Naughton, H.: The national exercise and heart disease project: report No. 2. Cardiology *62:* 352–367 (1978).
9 Strasser, T.: The WHO rehabilitation study; in Kellermann, Denolin, Critical evaluation of cardiac rehabilitation, pp. 174–176 (Karger, Basel 1977).
10 Froelicher, V. F.; Jensen, D.; Atwood, J. E.; Mckirnan, D.; Gerber, K.; Slutsky, R.; Battler, A.; Ashburn, W.; Ross, J.: Cardiac rehabilitation: evidence for improvement in myocardial perfusion and function. Archs. phys. Med. Rehabil. *61:* 517–522 (1980).
11 Feinstein, A. R.: Clinical biostatistics (Mosby, St. Louis 1977).
12 Cay, E. L.: Psychological problems in patients after a myocardial infarction; in Denolin, Psychological problems before and after myocardial infarction. Adv. Cardiol., vol. 29, pp. 108–112 (Karger, Basel 1982).

Jan J. Kellermann, MD, Cardiac Evaluation and Rehabilitation Institute,
Chaim Sheba Medical Center, 52621 Tel Hashomer (Israel)

Adv. Cardiol., vol. 31, pp. 138–141 (Karger, Basel 1982)

Early Ambulation: The Physiologic Basis Revisited[1]

Nanette K. Wenger

Emory University School of Medicine, Atlanta, Ga., USA

The pattern of care for patients with symptomatic coronary disease has changed markedly over the centuries. It is apparent from the writings of *Heberden, Parry, John Hunter,* and *Sir William McKenzie* that, during the 1700s and 1800s, the physical activity of coronary patients was not significantly limited. Indeed, the marked restriction of activity was a phenomenon of the 1920s–1940s; it followed the description of myocardial infarction and its consequences by *Herrick;* the data about pathologic anatomy from *Mallory, White,* and *Salcedo-Salgar,* and the subsequent clinical recommendations of *Sir Thomas Lewis* and *Jeter and White,* emphasizing that protracted strict bed rest was mandatory for the survival of patients with acute myocardial infarction. The current emphasis that the duration of bed rest could be safely decreased dated from the work and writings of *Levine, Dock, Harrison,* and *Stead and Warren* in the 1940s and 1950s. Actually, the emphasis of the late Dr. *Samuel Levine* was a preference for the sitting position (chair rest), designed to decrease venous return, rather than actual ambulation. Subsequent to that time, a number of controlled clinical trials in many countries throughout the world has documented the safety of early ambulation. Today's presentations further emphasized the feasibility, desirability and safety of the early ambulation approach for patients after myocardial infarction and after aortocoronary bypass surgery.

[1] Adapted from Wenger, N. K.: Early ambulation after myocardial infarction: rationale, program components, and results; in Wenger, Hellerstein, *Rehabilitation of the coronary patient* (Wiley, New York 1978).

Because of the general acceptance of this approach to care, the physiologic basis that underlies its application deserves review. Most of the rationale is based on the deleterious effects of prolonged bed-rest, and the documented advantages of early mobilization [1, 2].

The most marked alteration which occurs with prolonged bed rest is a decrease in physical work capacity. This is best illustrated by a study of the maximal oxygen uptake of healthy young college students, who were then placed at strict bed rest for 21 days; their physical work capacity was remeasured after the period at bed rest and subsequently serially while they participated in an exercise training program. The physical work capacity, as measured by exercise testing, decreased by 20–25% after 3weeks at bed rest, and at least 3weeks of training were required to restore the pre-bed-rest status. The higher the degree of physical fitness prior to bed rest, the longer the training required to return to the prior functional level after resumption of activity. Extrapolation of these data to the care of patients with symptomatic coronary disease identifies several important features. First, as illustrated by the sedentary and relatively unfit students, is the explanation of the paradoxic finding that sedentary patients after myocardial infarction, if they have not sustained major physiologic impairment, often can perform activities at a level greater than that prior to infarction when enrolled in an appropriate exercise training program. The second feature concerns the highly physically fit patient or one whose occupation requires heavy physical labor; these individuals decondition rapidly, and a far greater period of time, i.e. a greater intensity of training, is required to restore the pre-bed-rest status. Finally, the decrease in physical work capacity with immobilization raises serious question as to whether the post-illness fatigue and weakness commonly described in the patient at prolonged bed rest for myocardial infarction relates to the disease per se or to the therapy we have chosen to impose for the illness.

Additionally, clinicians are accustomed to encounter sinus tachycardia and orthostatic hypotension when a patient is initially mobilized after a period at bed-rest [3]. Neither response is desirable for the patient with recent myocardial infarction. Although the loss of normal postural vasomotor reflexes plays a role in these responses, they reflect primarily the hypovolemia of protracted bed rest; patients may sustain a decrease of as much as 700 or 800 cm^3 in their circulating blood volume within a week to 10 days at strict bed rest [4]. It is important to appreciate that activity as low level as allowing the patient to sit in a chair two or three times daily is adequate to avert the occurrence of hypovolemia and the resultant responses. It is equally interesting that patients with congestive heart failure, who obviously do not have a decreased circulating blood volume, do not manifest tachycardia and postural hypotension when they are mobilized after a period at bed rest [3]. An added concern is that when hypovolemia occurs, the plasma volume decreases to a greater extent than does the red blood cell mass [5], increasing blood viscosity and predisposing to thromboembolism; this problem is accentuated by the decreased use of the leg muscle pump at bed rest, which adds the thromboembolic risk of venous circulatory stasis to that of increased blood viscosity [6].

Pulmonary ventilation decreases modestly at bed rest, due to a decrease in lung volume and vital capacity; but this is probably significant only in the patient with associated chronic pulmonary disease. The negative nitrogen and protein balance [7, 8] which occurs at bed rest may potentially adversely affect the healing of a necrotic area of the myocardium and the formation of a small, firm, fibrous scar.

Finally, and of considerable consequence, is the decrease in skeletal muscle mass and muscular contractile strength and efficiency. Muscular contractile strength may decrease by 10% or 15% within the first week at bed rest. The problem is that inefficiently contracting muscle demands more oxygen, for any given task, and imposes this increased oxygen demand on an impaired oxygen transport system and potentially ischemic myocardium in the setting of acute infarction.

Several clinical applications of this have been elegantly presented to you during this symposium. Let me summarize, then, what we recognize as benefits to be anticipated from early ambulation of patients with myocardial infarction and after aortocoronary bypass surgery:

(1) a decrease in the deconditioning effects of protracted bed rest;

(2) a decrease in thromboembolic complications and pulmonary atelectasis;

(3) a decrease in emotional complications, particularly anxiety and depression;

(4) an improved functional capacity at the time of hospital discharge;

(5) enabling early exercise testing to be performed if desired;

(6) enabling a shorter hospitalization with its economic advantages and the potential for more optimal use of hospital beds, and

(7) because patients have become neither physically nor emotionally deconditioned, enabling an earlier and more complete return to work.

References

1 Saltin, B.; Blomqvist, G.; Mitchell, J. H. et al.: Response to exercise after bed rest and training. Circulation *37–38:* suppl. 7, p. 1 (1968).

2 Chobanian, A. V.; Little, R. D.; Tercyak, A. et al.: The metabolic and hemodynamic effects of prolonged bed rest in normal subjects. Circulation *49:* 551 (1974).

3 Fareeduddin, K.; Abelmann, W. H.: Impaired orthostatic intolerance after bed rest in patients with myocardial infarction. New Engl. J. Med. *280:* 345 (1969).

4 Hyatt, K. H.; Kamenetsky, L. G.; Smith, W. M.: Extravascular dehydration as an etiologic factor in post-recumbency orthostatism. Aerospace Med. *40:* 644 (1969).

5 Miller, P. B.; Johnson, R. L.; Lamp, L. E.: Effects of moderate physical exercise during four weeks of bed rest on circulatory functions in man. Aerospace Med. *36:* 1077 (1965).

6 Broustet, J. P.; Dubecq, M.; Bouloumie, J. et al.: Rehabilitation of the coronary patients: Mobilization program in the acute phase. Schweiz. med. Wschr. *103:* 57 (1973).

7 Lynch, T. N.; Jensen, R. L.; Stevens, P. M. et al.: Metabolic effects of prolonged bed rest: Their modification by simulated altitude. Aerospace Med. *38:* 10 (1967).

8 Deitrick, J. E.; Whedon, G. D.; Shorr, E.: Effects of immobilization upon various metabolic and physiologic functions of normal men. Am. J. Med. *4:* 3 (1948).

N. K. Wenger, MD, Emory University School of Medicine,
Thomas K. Glenn Memorial Building, 69 Butler Street, S. E., Atlanta, GA 30303 (USA)

Adv. Cardiol., vol. 31, pp. 142–146 (Karger, Basel 1982)

Complications during Early Ambulation and Patient Selection

J. A. Velasco, V. Tormo, F. Ridocci, A. Grima

Centro Valoración Funcional y Rehabilitación del Cardiaco,
Hospital Provincial, Valencia, Spain

Introduction

Appropriate selection of patients for early ambulation is mandatory. Some risk indicators may permit the physician to select the low-risk patients for early ambulation and discharge [1–3]. We have studied the complications presented by a group of myocardial infarction (MI) patients during their early ambulation at the general ward after they had been transferred from the CCU in order to find out whether these complications could be related with risk indicators noticed during the CCU stay (MI location, cardiac failure and arrhythmias) and some previous clinical data (age, sex, previous MI, diabetes and arterial hypertension).

Material and Methods

We studied retrospectively a group of 231 patients, selected from 383 who were admitted to our CCU during the period between January 1978 and March 1981 and diagnosed as having acute MI, following the WHO criteria for definite infarction [4]. The 231 patients were transferred from the CCU to the general ward of the Department of Cardiology 2–7 days after admission and all of them had experienced the first symptoms during the last 48 h before admission. The other 152 patients either were transferred to the general ward after the 7th day or admitted with a delay of more than 48 h and were excluded from the study. The number of days in the CCU was partly determined by the severity of the illness but also by the availability of beds at the general ward.

During their CCU stay, the patients made some passive and active movements of arms and legs and they also could wash hands and face and could seat up in bed. The usual contraindications for starting this early mobilization were considered: shock, cardiac failure, chest pain, temperature and arrhythmias.

On the first day after transfer to the general ward, the patients could sit in a chair and stand up; on the second day, they could walk to the bathroom. They started with low-intensity calisthenics and increased their caloric demands, following the WHO program [5], adapted and published by ourselves [6]. The program was either stopped or delayed when one of the following clinical signs was present: cardiac failure, malignant arrhythmias, persistent ST elevation, chest pain, dyspnea, decrease in systolic blood pressure, and heart rate more than 30 beats/min above the resting level during mobilization.

At the end of the first week in the general ward, the patients performed more intense dynamic calisthenics in two daily sessions of 10 min and during the second week they could climb stairs. Before discharge, all patients under 65 years of age performed an exercise test.

We studied the complications which appeared during the stay at the general ward: death, reinfarctions, cardiac failure and arrhythmias. In order to find out whether there was a correlation between these events and the clinical data, we studied the following data of each patient: age, sex, previous MI, arterial hypertension, diabetes, duration of the CCU stay, MI location, cardiac failure and arrhythmias observed during the CCU stay. The following signs of cardiac failure were considered: radiological lung edema, basal lung crepitations, third heart sound and breathlessness as well as the following arrhythmias: malignant VPBs (more frequent than 10%, multifocal, paired and early), ventricular tachycardia and fibrillation, atrial fibrillation and other frequent atrial arrhythmias.

Data analyses were performed using Student's t test.

Results

Patient Data

Of this group 88.3% were male and 11.7% female. The mean age was 59.8±12.3 years (range 31–83 years). The mean age of the women (66.5±7.8 years) was significantly higher ($p<0.0005$) than that of the men (59±11 years). 20 patients had suffered a previous MI (8.7%), 52 were hypertensive (22.5%) and 26 diabetic (11.3%).

CCU Stay

The mean duration of the CCU stay for the whole group of patients was 5.3±1.4 days (range 2–7 days). 56 patients (24.2%) remained at the CCU for 2–4 days and the rest (75.8%) stayed there for 5–7 days. 114 patients had an anterior wall MI (49.3%) and 117 an inferior wall MI (50.7%). 70 patients (30.3%) showed signs of cardiac failure during the CCU stay and 72 patients (31.2%) showed some of the arrhythmias studied. In spite of these clinical data the patients could be transferred to the general ward during the first 7 days.

Stay at the General Ward

The mean duration of the stay in the general ward was 11.3±4.2 days (range 6–30 days). During this time, 15 patients died of their cardiac illness

(6.5%): 5 patients died suddenly (during the first 2 h after the onset of symptoms), 5 died of a reinfarction, 4 of acute left-ventricular failure and 1 of thromboembolism. All reinfarctions were fatal and the signs of cardiac failure appeared in 29 cases (12.5%); 22 (75.8%) of these patients had shown the same signs during the CCU stay. Arrhythmias appeared in 14 patients (6.1%), 10 of them (71.2%) showed the rhythm disturbances during the acute phase. In the group of patients who died there were 8 cases (52%), without cardiac failure and arrhythmias during the stay at the general ward. On the other hand, 73.3% of the patients who died showed these complications during the CCU stay. The identification of these complications during the CCU stay is useful for detecting patients at risk during the ambulation program.

Cardiac Mortality during Early Ambulation

During the stay at the general ward, 15 patients (6.5%) died of cardiac illness. The mortality rate was higher in females (4/27; 14.8%) than in males (11/204; 5.4%) and the difference was significant ($p<0.05$). The cardiac mortality was highly age-dependent: there was no mortality case among patients under 55 years of age, the rate was of 2.6% (2/78) among patients between 55 and 65 years; it was much higher (16.7%) among patients over 65 years of age (13/78). These differences were highly significant ($p<0.002$).

The higher mortality rate in females seemed to be age-dependent: their mean age (66.4 years) was significantly higher ($p<0.0005$) than that of males (59 years). Nevertheless, the females showed a higher prevalence of arterial hypertension (62.9%) and diabetes (18.5%) than the males (17.2 and 10.3%, respectively). The rest of the data – previous MI, MI location, cardiac failure and arrhythmias – showed a similar frequency in both sexes.

The mortality rate was not significantly different in patients with a previous MI (15%), arterial hypertension (5.8%) and diabetes (no case of death). This low mortality rate in patients with diabetes or arterial hypertension supports the conclusion that the high mortality rate in females was related only to the age. There was no difference in mortality in relation to the duration of the CCU stay (less than 4 days: 7.1%; 5–7 days: 6.3%) and to the MI location (anterior wall MI: 7.9%; inferior wall MI: 5.1%).

On the other hand, patients who showed cardiac failure during their CCU stay and patients with arrhythmias had higher mortality rates (12.9%, 9/70, and 15.3%, 11/72, respectively). Both of these rates were statistically significantly higher than the total mortality rate (6.5%) of the group ($p<0.05$ and $p<0.01$, respectively). Only 3 patients without cardiac failure and arrhythmias died during their stay at the general ward (2.6%).

Identification of High-Risk Patients

Comparing the group of 15 patients who died with the 216 patients who were alive on discharge, there were significant differences in relation to the age of both groups (72.3 ± 8.4 vs. 59.2 ± 11.7 years; $p<0.0005$) and in relation to the proportion of females (26.6 vs. 10%; $p<0.05$). Nevertheless, this higher proportion of females in the group who died is highly dependent on age, as we showed previously.

The presence of cardiac failure and arrhythmias during the CCU stay was also significantly higher in the group of patients who died (cardiac failure 60% and arrhythmias 73%) than in the survivors (27% in both cases) and both differences were statistically significant ($p<0.01$ and $p<0.002$, respectively).

On the other hand there were no differences in both groups in relation to previous MI, arterial hypertension, diabetes, duration of CCU stay and MI location.

Discussion

It is necessary to select high-risk patients before early ambulation. *Chaturvedi* et al. [2] excluded patients with arrhythmias, tachycardia, ST segment elevation and chest pain, and *Hays* et al. [3] those patients with angina, cardiac failure and arrhythmias. An ad hoc committee [7] recommended the exclusion of patients with ischemia in evolution, left-ventricular failure, shock, severe arrhythmias and conduction disturbances.

Royston [8], in a report similar to ours, found a different mortality rate related to the presence of arrhythmias during the CCU stay and to the age. *Bloch* et al. [9] found also a higher mortality rate before discharge among patients who were excluded from the program because of complications during the CCU stay. *Lindvall* et al. [1] proved that the mortality rate was related to some risk indicators and that patients without those risk indicators could safely be discharged on the 9th day after MI.

Following our results and those of the literature we can conclude that it is necessary to select patients before starting them on an early ambulation program. In our study group, we found that patients over 65 years of age and those with cardiac failure or arrhythmias during the acute phase are at a higher risk and must be excluded from such a program.

References

1 Lindvall, K.; Erhardt, L. R.; Lundman, T.; Rehnyrist, N.; Sjögren, A.: Early mobilization and discharge of patients with acute myocardial infarction. Acta med. scand. *206:* 169–175 (1979).

2 Chaturvedi, N. C.; Walsh, M. J.; Evans, A.; Munro, P.; Boyle, Mc C.; Barber, J. M.: Selection of patients for early discharge after acute myocardial infarction. Br. Heart J. *36:* 533–535 (1974).

3 Hays, M. J.; Morris, G. K.; Hampton, J. R.: Comparison of mobilization after two and nine days in uncomplicated myocardial infarction. Br. med. J. *iii:* 10–13 (1974).

4 World Health Organization: Evaluation of comprehensive rehabilitative and preventive programmes for patients after acute myocardial infarction. Report on two working groups. EURO 8206(8) (WHO, Regional Office for Europe, Copenhagen 1973).

5 World Health Organization: A program for the physical rehabilitation of patients with acute myocardial infarction (WHO, Regional Office for Europe, Copenhagen 1968).

6 Tormo Alfonso, V.; Velasco Rami, J. A.: Valoración funcional y rehabilitación de la cardiopatía coronaria, pp. 291–301 (Edit. Médica y Técnica, Barcelona 1978).

7 Swan, H. J. C.; Blackburn, H. W.; de Sanctis, R.; Frommer, P. L.; Hurst, J. W.; Paulo, O.; Rapaport, E.; Wallace, A.; Weinberg, S.: Duration of hospitalization in uncomplicated completed acute myocardial infarction. An ad hoc committee review. Am. J. Cardiol. *37:* 413–419 (1976).

8 Royston, G. R.: Short stay hospital treatment and rapid rehabilitation of cases of myocardial infarction in a district hospital. Br. Heart J. *34:* 526–532 (1972).

9 Bloch, A.; Maeder, J. P.; Haisly, J. C.; Felix, J.; Blackburn, H.: Early mobilization after myocardial infarction. A controlled study. Am. J. Cardiol. *34:* 152–157 (1974).

J. A. Velasco, MD, Centro Valoración Funcional y Rehabilitación del Cardiaco, Hospital Provincial, Valencia (Spain)

Adv. Cardiol., vol. 31, pp. 147–151 (Karger, Basel 1982)

Early Ambulation after Myocardial Infarction

The Surgical Model

Robert M. Kohn[1]

Buffalo General Hospital, Buffalo, N.Y., USA

It seems strange that in the 1980s we continue to debate the dangers and merits of early ambulation for the patient with myocardial infarction. In 1975, at a Rehabilitation section meeting in Tel Aviv and subsequently at other international meetings [1, 2], we discussed the definitions and semantics of early mobilization, the psychologic benefits, the economic benefits, and we bemoaned the lack of long-term follow-up studies. At the time of the 1975 meeting, I pointed out the lack of information on staging of myocardial infarctions for rehabilitation potential, and the inadequate information on subgroup analysis to identify those for whom it would be safe to mobilize on day 1 or 2, versus those who might benefit from prolonged rest [3]. Since then these areas still remain largely unreported.

I believe there is general agreement today that, if early arrhythmias are controlled, prognosis after a myocardial infarction is a function of the amount of myocardial damage. The patient left with congestive heart failure or enlarged heart is more arrhythmia-prone, and there is no evidence that prolonging rest alters his outcome.

With the advent of coronary artery bypass surgery we have had the opportunity to observe patients who routinely are ambulated early. Many of these patients have suffered perioperative myocardial infarctions, some identified only in retrospect.

At the Buffalo General Hospital we have analyzed the experience of 319 consecutive open heart surgical cases, from January through September of 1981. Criteria for diagnosing intraoperative myocardial infarction

[1] The author is indebted to Dr. *Syed Raza* and Ms. *Betsey Gehring* for assistance in obtaining the surgical data.

Table I. Criteria

Q:	Not previously present in lead Amplitude at least 2mm and duration 0.03 s or more
	Disappearance of, or diminution amplitude R any V lead, providing R present and taller in leads to left and right
ST:	Reciprocal changes 1 and 3 and/or AVL and AVF 1mm or more

Table II. MI by ECG (total reviewed 319)

Definite MI	59
Probable	4
Extension	1
	64
Complicated (deaths 8)	23
Favorable results	41

were limited to the electrocardiogram, since the attachment to the pump and the surgery itself usually cause significant rises of cardiac enzymes.

Criteria for electrocardiographic diagnosis of infarction are given in table I. New Q waves were defined as the appearance of a significant Q according to the Minnesota Code that had not been observed in preoperative electrocardiograms in those leads. A significant Q_3 required the presence of a new Q in either lead 2 or aVL in addition. The majority of the patients showed evidence of pericarditis (or injury current from cold cardioplegia) manifested by global ST elevation in the first 48 h of their postoperative period. These changes were ignored in the classification. Reciprocal ST changes were classified as criteria for new infarction only in the limb leads. Those with left bundle branch block, or those with pacemakers could not be classified electrocardiographically and were excluded from the analysis.

Using the above criteria it was possible to identify 59 definite and 4 probable new infarctions and 1 extention of a preoperative infarction in patients undergoing various types of open heart surgery (table II).

Routine postoperative orders after such open heart surgery include sitting in a chair as soon as extubated (usually within 12 h of completion of

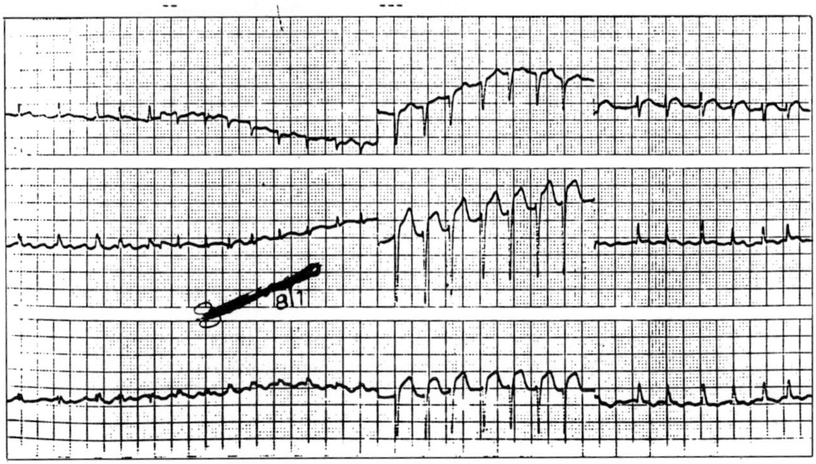

Fig. 1.

surgery), and walking to the bathroom and to the treatment room for pulmonary exercises to encourage lung re-expansion at 48 h post operation after removal of chest tubes. Rhythm is routinely monitored only for the first 24–48 h. By the 5th postoperative day the patients are doing mild exercises and by the 7th postoperative day are either discharged or transferred to an active rehabilitation program.

Exceptions to the above were 23 patients who required prolonged inotropic support, and had cerebral complications, sepsis, or respiratory complications. 8 of these patients died, only 4 from pump failure secondary to the infarction. Five of the deaths were on postoperative days 1 through 4 prior to attempts to ambulate, and 3 were late deaths, only one related to the heart.

The diagnosis of intraoperative infarction was usually made on electrocardiograms recorded postoperatively on days 1, 2 and 3 and compared with preoperative tracings. Clinically, they were interpreted within 24 h after the recording. Retrospective review of the electrocardiograms and their re-reading to indentify infarcts according to the criteria outlined above showed that the diagnosis of new infarction was often not included in the original interpretation of the routine ECG reading.

There was no significant difference in the short- or long-term results of those surviving intraoperative infarcts as compared to those who did not experience this complication. There is not a single identified instance of myocardial rupture in those who died after having transmural intraopera-

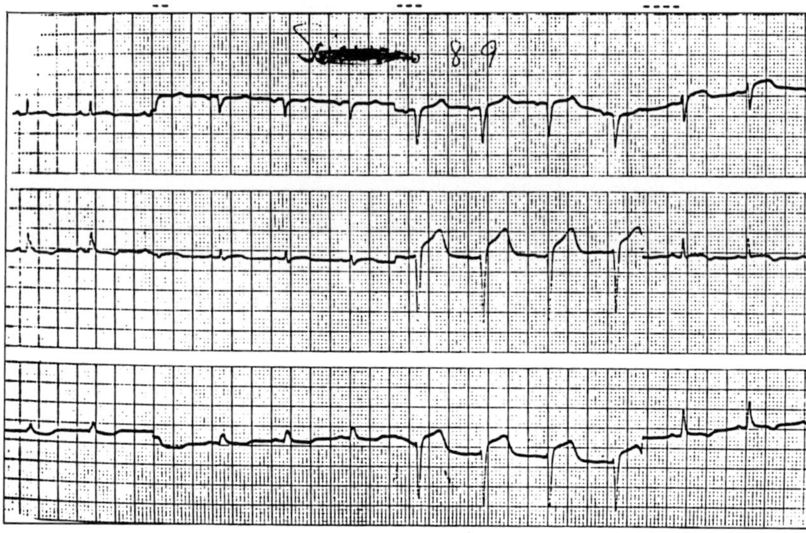

Fig. 2.

tive myocardial infarctions. When a perioperative infarction was identified, the management was not different from that of the uncomplicated group.

As an anecdotal illustration, a 56-year-old lawyer with chest pain on exertion or exposure to cold and an abnormal exercise test at 4 METs with pain reproduced, had a coronary angiogram showing 90% occlusion of LAD artery proximal to any branching. His resting preoperative ECG is shown in figure 1. 24 h after bypass he had atrial fibrillation, rales in his chest, and an ECG as shown in figure 2. After digitalis, the next day his ECG was as shown in figure 3, and since then has shown QS in V_1 through V_3 and a qR in V_4. He showed no further evidence of congestive failure and was ambulated at 48 h as if nothing had happened. He was unaware of any problems. He has been free of angina and failure and at full activity for the past year.

For the coronary artery bypass graft patient, the experience in Buffalo is that survival is exactly the same over a 5-year period as those of the same age and sex who never had any knowledge of heart disease [4].

If early ambulation in the presence of myocardial infarction is so well tolerated by the surgical patients, it is difficult to see why we continue to agonize over the problem for the non-surgically induced myocardial infarction patient.

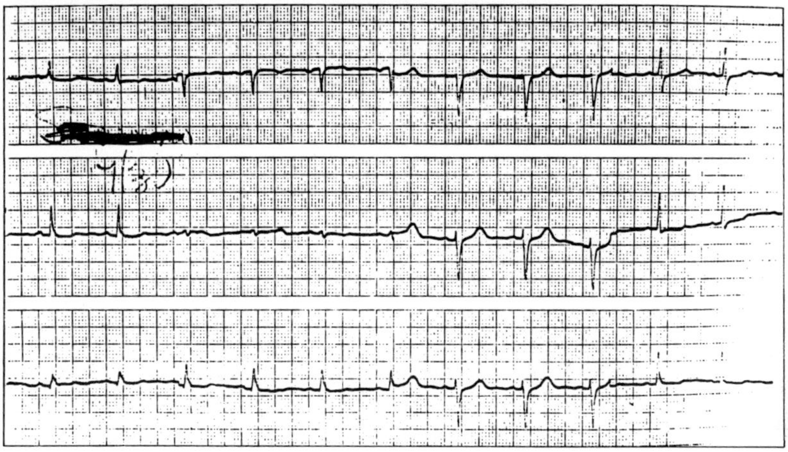

Fig. 3.

In both groups rhythm is monitored for the initial 48 h. The rhythm can be monitored whether the patient is in bed, in a chair, or on a commode. In the absence of pump failure patients can be safely ambulated. Let us individualize care, but refrain from overprotecting by abusing bed rest.

References

1 Kellermann, J.; Denolin, H.: Critical evaluation of cardiac rehabilitation. Biblthca cardiol., No. 36 (Karger, Basel 1976).

2 Raineri, A.; Kellermann, J.; Rulli, V.: Selected topics in exercise cardiology and rehabilitation (Plenum Press, New York 1980).

3 Kohn, R.: A critique of ambulation studies. Biblthca cardiol., No. 36, pp. 62–66 (Karger, Basel 1976).

4 Greene, D.; et al.: Long-term survival after coronary bypass surgery. Br. Heart J. *45:* 417–426 (1981).

Prof. R. M. Kohn, Buffalo General Hospital, Heart Station, Buffalo, NY 14203 (USA)

Adv. Cardiol., vol. 31, pp. 152–155 (Karger, Basel 1982)

Accelerated versus Classical Early Mobilization after Myocardial Infarction

R. Messin, B. Demaret

Department of Cardiology, University Hospital Saint-Pierre, Brussels, Belgium

During the last years, there has been an increasing tendency to accelerate the process of physical reconditioning during the acute phase (phase I) of myocardial infarction [1–7]. This has led to a significant reduction of the mean hospitalization duration in the coronary care unit which, in our department, has shifted from about 2 weeks to 10–12 days. (Provided, of course, that there are no major complications like sustained angina, severe arrhythmias, heart failure, or any inflammatory process).

The purpose of the present study is to compare the outcome of two groups of patients with myocardial infarction, both being treated in our coronary care unit after randomized selection.

Material and Methods

The control group consisted of 49 patients without major complications who were submitted to a rehabilitation program, physical training starting on the 2nd day and going on through three stages. Walking was allowed on the 8th day and discharge from hospital took place after 2 weeks. Thereafter, a training program was pursued at home, during the early convalescence period (phase II), through four stages of increasing intensity and duration. Climbing stairs, in particular, was generally allowed 3 weeks after the acute attack. A complete functional evaluation was then performed after 2 months and a follow-up was organized 1 year later.

The intervention group consisted of 49 patients without major complications who were submitted to a more accelerated mobilization program, walking starting on the 5th day instead on the 8th day. A submaximal exercise test was performed on the 10th day; if no complications occurred, climbing stairs was allowed on the next day instead in the 4th week. In this group, too, a complete functional evaluation was performed 2 months after the acute attack and a follow-up was settled 1 year later.

The two groups were quite comparable before entering the study:

(1) All patients were males.

(2) The age distribution was the same in the two groups, the highest frequency lying between 50 and 59 years. No statistically significant difference could be detected by the χ^2 test.

(3) The location of myocardial infarction showed no statistically significant difference between the two groups, 33 % anterior and 53 % inferior location in the intervention group compared to 39 and 49 % in the control group, plus some combined or more exceptional locations.

(4) The clinical evolution was similar in the two groups during their stay in the coronary care unit, with 37 % of ventricular and 14 % of supraventricular arrhythmias in the intervention group compared to 26 and 18 % in the control group, 4 % of conduction disturbances and 4 % of reduced ventricular function in the intervention group compared to 8 and 2 % in the control group.

(5) A retrospective analysis of the kinds of professional activities performed before the coronary attack was also performed: work was light in 27 %, moderate in 43, and heavy in 14 % of the cases in the intervention group compared to 31, 45 and 12 % in the control group. About 16 % were not working before the myocardial infarction in the intervention group compared to 12 % in the control group. Also here no statistical difference was to be found between the two groups.

Results

2 months after the acute phase all patients were submitted to a multistage maximal exercise test on the bicycle ergometer, and the physical working capacity was compared. A low capacity (≤50 W) was less frequent in the intervention group (4 % compared to 12 % in the control group), while a high capacity (100 W, ≥125 W) was more frequent (63 % compared to 35 %); the difference between the two distributions was statistically significant at the 5 % level. 37 % of the cases stopped the test owing to electrocardiographical or clinical signs of coronary insufficiency in the intervention group compared to 43 % in the control group; the difference was not significant.

A follow-up study was performed in all cases 1 year after myocardial infarction, and informations were collected concerning (1) the return to professional work and (2) morbidity and mortality.

(1) 57 % of the patients returned to their professional activities in the intervention group compared to 39 % in the control group. These figures suggest some differences between the two groups, although the probability level lies between 10 and 25 %, being not significant from a statistical point of view. The remaining patients of both groups were pensioned, invalids or dead; no follow-up could be obtained in a few percent of cases belonging to the control group.

(2) Concerning morbidity and mortality, 16% of the patients of the intervention group had a reinfarction within 1 year and 8% died; reinfarction was proved to be the cause of death in 50% of the cases. In the control group, 4% had a reinfarction and only 2% died. The latter percentage corresponds to 1 patient who had a cerebrovascular attack. The difference was statistically significant at the 5% level.

Conclusions

This limited study suggests several remarks:

(1) Accelerated early mobilization of the patients after myocardial infarction without major complications is harmless; in particular, it does not enhance supraventricular or ventricular arrhythmias.

(2) The advantage of accelerated early mobilization is that the patients are resuming rather heavy physical activities like climbing stairs while they are still under the supervision of the medical staff of the coronary care unit, instead of being at home where no close control is available.

(3) Accelerated early mobilization makes it possible to reduce the length of hospitalization in the coronary care unit to about 10–12 days and, thus, to accelerate the turnover of patients which can be beneficial from an economical point of view.

(4) The results suggest that there would be a tendency in patients who underwent accelerated early mobilization to be, later on, more often professionally rehabilitated.

(5) Nevertheless, a drawback of accelerated early mobilization seems to be a higher rate of reinfarction and death after 1 year follow-up. One reason could be that, although those patients are physically more fit than the control group and psychologically well motivated to return to their professional activities, the physiological and mental stress that such activities imply have a deleterious influence on the long-term prognosis of coronary disease.

References

1 Abraham, A. S.; Sever, Y.; Weinstein, M.; Dollberg, M.; Menczel, J.: Value of early ambulation in patients with and without complications after acute myocardial infarction. New Engl. J. Med. *292:* 719 (1975).

2 Bloch, A.; Maeder, J. P.; Haissly, J. C.; Felix, J.; Blackburn, H.: Early mobilization after myocardial infarction. Am. J. Cardiol. *34:* 152 (1974).
3 Hayes, M. J.; Morris, G. K.; Hampton, J. R.: Comparison of mobilization after two and nine days in uncomplicated myocardial infarction. Br. Heart J. *36:* 10 (1974).
4 McNeer, J. F.; Wallace, A. G.; Wagner, G. S.; Starmer, C. F.; Rosati, R. A.: The course of acute myocardial infarction. Feasibility of early discharge of the uncomplicated patient. Circulation *51:* 410 (1975).
5 Miller, A. J.: Rehabilitation and length of hospitalization after acute myocardial infarction. Am. Heart J. *92:* 547 (1976).
6 Swan, H. J. C.; Blackburn, H. W.; Sanctis, R. de; Frommer, P. L.; Hurst, J. W.; Paul, O.; Rapaport, E.; Wallace, A.; Weinberg, S.: Duration of hospitalization in 'uncomplicated completed acute myocardial infarction'. Am. J. Cardiol. *37:* 413 (1976).
7 Thornley, P. E.; Turner, R. W. D.: Rapid mobilization after acute myocardial infarction. First step in rehabilitation and secondary prevention. Br. Heart J. *39:* 471 (1977).

Roger Messin, Department of Cardiology, University Hospital Saint-Pierre,
322, rue Haute, B-1000 Brussels (Belgium)

Adv. Cardiol., vol. 31, pp. 156–161 (Karger, Basel 1982)

Physical Conditioning Following Myocardial Infarction

Robert F. DeBusk

Stanford University School of Medicine, Stanford, Calif., USA

In performing treadmill exercise testing at regular intervals following clinically uncomplicated myocardial infarction [1] we noted a sizable increase in functional capacity between 3 and 11 weeks following the acute event even in patients who underwent no formal reconditioning during this interval: functional capacity increased from 7.0±1.9 to 9.7±1.8 METs or multiples of resting energy expenditure. In order to evaluate the mechanisms responsible for this spontaneous improvement in functional capacity and to determine the extent to which it could be augmented by physical reconditioning, we studied 70 men with a mean age of 54±3 years [2]. Following symptom-limited treadmill exercise testing 3 weeks after infarction, these men were randomly assigned to undergo 8 weeks of exercise conditioning at home (n = 12) or in a gymnasium environment (n = 28) or were given no formal instructions for physical activity (control patients, n = 30). Patients participating in exercise conditioning at home or in a gymnasium underwent 3 h per week of continuous bicycle exercise or jogging at individually prescribed heart rates between 95 and 115 beats/minute during the first 4 weeks and between 110 and 125 beats/minute during the second 4 weeks.

11 weeks after infarction, values of peak functional capacity were significantly greater in men who had undergone training in the gymnasium or at home than in those who did not receive formal reconditioning: 11.0±1.6, 10.3±1.4 and 9.4±1.8 METs, respectively ($p<0.05$). These values of functional capacity were similar to those of sedentary men of similar age without coronary heart disease and would not have limited their capacity to perform vocational and avocational activities 7 weeks or sooner following myocardial infarction.

The higher functional capacity in the gymnasium training group than in the control group was limited to patients who did not demonstrate exercise-induced ischemic ST-segment depression or angina pectoris during treadmill exercise testing at 3 or 11 weeks following infarction. In other words, the greatest increase in functional capacity noted in patients undergoing gymnasium training occurred in those whose lack of ischemic response and consequent better prognosis might have enabled them to carry out an equivalent amount of exercise in a nonsupervised setting. Patients who were given no formal recommendations for physical activity were physically active 3–11 weeks following infarction: they reported walking 1.8–2.9 miles per day during this interval. The substantial improvement in functional capacity noted in these patients and their attainment at 11 weeks of values of functional capacity approximating those of normal sedentary men suggested that even low level physical effort such as walking might bestow substantial physical benefits in patients recovering from myocardial infarction. It appeared that these patients were more physically active than they would have been had they not undergone treadmill testing.

It therefore appeared important to evaluate the effects of treadmill exercise testing separate from those of exercise training in patients recovering from myocardial infarction. Accordingly, we have undertaken a separate study involving 60 men with clinically uncomplicated myocardial infarction with a mean age of 54±6 years. These patients were randomized into five groups 3 weeks after infarction: Group I ($n = 15$) had no treadmill testing until 6 months after infarction and did not undergo training during this interval, group II ($n = 8$) had testing but no training, group IIIA ($n = 20$) had testing and up to 6 months of home training and group IIIB ($n = 17$) had testing and up to 6 months of gymnasium training. Treadmill testing was performed in all but group I patients at 11 weeks and in all patients at 6 months. Training consisted of walking, jogging or stationary cycling for 3 h per week. The electrocardiograms of patients performing home training were transmitted by a transtelephonic device to a monitoring station during exercise twice weekly. No complications of treadmill testing or of exercise training were noted. During the first 6 months following infarction, group II men who performed exercise testing only reported higher physical activity levels than group I men who did not undergo treadmill testing until 6 months after infarction. Compliance to both home and gymnasium training regimens was high. At 6 months, peak functional capacity in groups I, II, IIIA and IIIB was 7.5±1.9*, 8.3±2.2, 8.7±1.3 and 8.6±1.6 METs, respectively (*$p < 0.03$ versus other groups).

This experience suggested that functional capacity at 6 months was higher in patients undergoing treadmill exercise testing at 3 weeks than in those who did not perform treadmill testing until 6 months, whether or not patients underwent formal exercise training during this interval. Treadmill testing 3 weeks after infarction appeared to enhance functional capacity by encouraging a return to usual activities. Home training and gymnasium training appeared equally effective in augmenting functional capacity in these postinfarction patients.

What are the mechanisms responsible for the increased functional capacity following infarction, even in patients who undergo no formal reconditioning? Improvement in left ventricular function assessed by gated cardiac blood pool scanning does not appear to account for the improvement in functional capacity noted in our patients 1–11 weeks after infarction, whether or not they have undergone formal exercise conditioning during this interval. For example, in 38 men with a mean age of 55±4 years, ejection fraction at rest was similar at 7, 21 and 77 days following clinically uncomplicated myocardial infarction: 41, 47 and 49%, respectively. At a relatively constant bicycle workload of 450–1500 kg/minute and exercise heart rate of 118–124 beats/minute ejection fraction was 57, 54 and 53% at 7, 21 and 77 days, respectively [2].

Regression of myocardial ischemia as assessed by thallium myocardial perfusion imaging does not appear to account for the spontaneous improvement in functional capacity which occurs 1–11 weeks following infarction. In the 38 postinfarction men described above, the incidence of reversibly ischemic thallium defects at 7, 21 and 77 days was 19, 33 and 38%, a difference which was not statistically significant [3].

These data indicate that changes in 'central' cardiac performance related to left ventricular dysfunction and myocardial ischemia do not appear to account for the spontaneous improvement in functional capacity noted 1–11 weeks after myocardial infarction.

We considered that 'peripheral' changes related to bedrest and physical inactivity might contribute to the relatively low functional capacity measured 1–3 weeks following infarction and to the large spontaneous increase in functional capacity noted during the subsequent 8 weeks. In order to evaluate the contribution of bedrest deconditioning to the decrease in functional capacity noted in postinfarction patients, we studied 12 normal men with a mean age of 50±4 years who underwent 10 days' bedrest – an interval similar to that commonly encountered by middle-aged patients recovering from myocardial infarction [4]. These normal subjects performed symptom-limited upright and supine bicycle ergometry at baseline and after 10 days' bedrest. Following bedrest, left ventricular volume during supine rest diminished by 17% ($p<0.05$) compared to prebedrest values, functional capacity during *upright* exercise declined by 15% ($p<0.05$) but during *supine* exercise the decline was only 6% (n.s.).

Heart rate at rest and during submaximal exercise in the upright position increased following bedrest ($p<0.05$) whereas heart rate at rest and during exercise in the supine position did not change significantly.

Left ventricular ejection fraction was measured by gated cardiac blood pool scanning. Following bedrest, values of resting left ventricular ejection fraction were 0.75±0.08 and 0.77±0.13 in the supine and upright positions, respectively, and increased to 0.84±0.12 and 0.85±0.11 during near-maximal effort. Regional contraction abnormalities were not observed during pre- or postbedrest supine or upright effort.

The fact that functional capacity declined significantly during upright but not during supine effort following bedrest indicated that orthostatic factors and not ventricular dysfunction or physical inactivity were primarily responsible for the decline in functional capacity following bedrest. Peak oxygen consumption during upright exercise fell because even a substantial increase in heart rate and in ejection fraction were unable to compensate for the inadequate cardiac preload resulting from pooling of blood in the lower extremities following bedrest.

Strategies to limit the decrease in functional capacity following myocardial infarction have emphasized formal exercise reconditioning but simple exposure to gravitational stress substantially accomplishes this purpose [5]. In contrast, even vigorous supine exercise training fails to *prevent* the deteriorative effects of bedrest on peak oxygen consumption [6]. It appears that the deterioration of oxygen transport capacity resulting from bedrest may be largely obviated by gravitational stress such as intermittent sitting or standing, whereas formal physical reconditioning may fail to accomplish this purpose [7].

We evaluated the effects of formal exercise reconditioning in the 12 normal middle-aged men who had undergone 10 days of bedrest. Half of the subjects were randomly allocated to undergo a program of vigorous bicycle exercise training during 60 days after bedrest and 6 men resumed their usual prebedrest activities. 30 days' postbedrest values of peak oxygen consumption in training and in control men were not significantly different from prebedrest values: 24.7±4.6 and 26.4±6.4 ml/kg/min, respectively [8]. It appeared that resumption of habitual physical activity for 30 days after bedrest was as effective as formal exercise training in restoring peak oxygen consumption to prebedrest values. The fact that all subjects regained their prebedrest levels of functional capacity at approximately the same time appears to reflect the reversal of bedrest-induced decline in intravascular and cardiac volume.

Taken together, these data in postinfarction patients and in normal middle-aged subjects indicate the importance of a bedrest-induced decline in intravascular volume in limiting exercise tolerance and the importance of gravitational stresses in restoring exercise tolerance following bedrest.

The spontaneous improvement in functional capacity following myocardial infarction appears to reflect an important additional factor of a spontaneous increase in maximal heart rate, unaccompanied by significant improvement in ventricular function or in myocardial perfusion. We noted a significant increase in peak heart rate between 3 and 7 weeks following infarction even in patients in whom an inadequate effort on the first visit was excluded: functional capacity on the second of two tests performed at 3 and at 7 weeks after infarction was no higher than on the first test [1]. The increase in peak heart rate from approximately 135 to 150 beats/minute appeared to account for most of the increase in functional capacity observed 3 and 7 weeks following infarction.

Strategies to deal with improvement in functional capacity following myocardial infarction should emphasize low level physical activity such as walking. The extent to which more vigorous exercise conditioning in either a home or a gymnasium environment will further augment functional capacity in such patients remains to be demonstrated.

In the final analysis, the success of rehabilitative efforts depends on the ability to define and improve three major areas of functioning: prognosis, functional capacity and psychosocial status. Exercise testing performed soon after myocardial infarction effectively addresses these issues: (1) It provides the physician and the patient with a realistic appraisal of the prognosis [9, 10] and of the need for further diagnostic evaluation and medical or surgical therapy. (2) It provides individualized guidelines for physical activity commencing soon after the acute event, at a time when patients manifest concern about the safety of physical exercise. (3) By reducing the patient's medically unwarranted concerns with prognosis and physical activity, it obviates much of the psychosocial distress which follows myocardial infarction. The simplicity and widespread availability of exercise testing may greatly increase the effectiveness of the physician in meeting the physical and psychosocial needs of patients recovering from myocardial infarction.

References

1 Haskell, W.; DeBusk, R.: Cardiovascular responses to repeated treadmill exercise testing soon after myocardial infarction. Circulation *60:* 1247–1251 (1979).

2 DeBusk, R.; et al.: Exercise training soon after myocardial infarction. Am. J. Cardiol. *44:* 1223–1229 (1979).

3 Hung, et al.: The effects of exercise training on myocardial ischemic and left ventricular function soon after myocardial infarction: a randomized study. Circulation *64:* suppl. (in press).

4 Convertino, et al.: Cardiovascular responses to exercise in middle-aged men following ten days of bedrest. Circulation (in press).

5 Convertino, V. A.; Sandler, H.; Webb, P.: The effect of an elastic reverse gradient garment on the cardiorespiratory deconditioning following 15 days bed rest. Aerospace Med. Ass. Preprinats. *148:* (1978).

6 Birkhead N. C.; et al.: Cardiodynamic and metabolic effects of prolonged bed rest with daily recombent or sitting exercise and with sitting inactivity. Tech. Rep. No. AMRL-TDR-64-61, p. 1 (Wright-Patterson Air Force Base, Ohio 1964).

7 Sivarajan, et al.: In-hospital exercise after myocardial infarction does not improve treadmill performance. New Engl. J. Med. *305:* 357–362 (1981).

8 DeBusk, R.; et al.: Randomized trial of exercise training following bedrest in normal middle-aged men: relevance to patients recovering from myocardial infarction. Clin. Res. (in press).

9 Markiewicz, W.; Houston, N.; DeBusk, R. F.: Exercise testing soon after myocardial infarction. Circulation *56:* 26–31 (1977).

10 Theroux, et al.: Prognostic value of exercise testing soon after myocardial infarction. New Engl. J. Med. *301:* 341–345 (1979).

R. F. DeBusk, MD, Cardiac Rehabilitation Program, Stanford University School of Medicine, 730 Welch Road, Suite B, Palo Alto, CA 94304 (USA)

Adv. Cardiol., vol. 31, pp. 162–167 (Karger, Basel 1982)

Primary Coronary Risk Factors and Secondary Prevention of Coronary Heart Disease

M. Kornitzer

Laboratory of Epidemiology and Social Medicine, Free University of Brussels, Belgium

Introduction

Three primary coronary risk factors have been repeatedly found to be involved in the incidence of coronary heart disease (CHD): hypercholesterolemia, high blood pressure, and cigarette smoking. All three were also observed to predict recurrence of myocardial infarction (MI), that is, to be secondary risk factors, although their predictive power is much weaker [2].

In the Coronary Drug Project (CDP), the risk ratio of recurrent MI or sudden death (SD) for subjects with high versus low serum cholesterol was around 1.5, whereas we observed a relative risk for first MI (fatal or nonfatal) or SD of 2.3 in subjects free of CHD at entry in a 10-year Belgian incidence study [8]. Notwithstanding the small gradient observed in MI subjects, the absolute excess risk associated with high serum cholesterol is much larger than in subjects without CHD; hence, if a decrease of serum cholesterol would be associated with a decrease in MI, the observed gain should be larger, compared to that in primary prevention. Randomized controlled trials in the secondary prevention of MI have only been performed in relation to serum cholesterol, and the least one can say is that they gave conflicting results.

Secondary prevention through diet was started more than 20 years ago, as can be seen from the study of *Morrison* [12] (table I): in a low-fat nonrandomized, but controlled study all patients in the control group were dead after 12 years. A collaborative group did not observe a significant reduction in recurrent MI [19]. The same was true for the study of *Rose* et al. [20] as well as for the soybean study [17]. The only important study with significant positive results was published by *Leren* [9]. He observed a

Table I. Secondary prevention: diet

Reference	n	Diet	Results
12	100	low fat	significant reduction in mortality (12 years)
19	264	low fat	nonsignificant reduction in fatal and nonfatal MI
20	80	low fat + corn oil	nonsignificant increase in fatal and nonfatal MI (2 years)
9	412	low fat + soybean oil	significant reduction in fatal and nonfatal MI
17	393	low fat + soybean oil	nonsignificant difference

significant reduction in fatal and nonfatal MI in the treated group after 5 years follow-up.

The most important randomized controlled trial on lipid-lowering drugs was the CDP [3–6] (table II). Not one single drug used in that study was able to reduce the CHD mortality: estrogens and dextrothyroxine had even an iatrogenic effect! In fact, the estrogen story started 20 years ago, when the groups of *Marmorston* et al. [10] and *Stamler* et al. [23] published the results of controlled trials in secondary prevention. The *Stamler* group randomized 275 MI patients, the treatment group receiving 5 mg estrogens. The 5-year mortality rates were reduced by about 50 % or more by hormone treatment. *Marmorston* et al. [10] randomized patients recovering from an acute MI. 147 of them received a placebo, 120 received ethinyl estradiol, and 85 received premarin (conjugated equine estrogens). Whereas ethinyl estradiol did not improve survival, this was the case for subjects receiving conjugated equine estrogens (premarin).

The Veterans Administration Cooperative Urological Research Group [24] published interesting results concerning a randomized trial of the treatment of patients with cancer of the prostate. More than 2,000 patients were enrolled. The group concluded: although estrogen therapy (5 mg) causes a modest decrease in the mortality from prostatic cancer, this decrease is outweighted by a substantial elevation in the mortality from other causes, primarily heart disease and cerebrovascular accidents. Coming back to the CDP study, it should be noted that clofibrate (1.8 g/day) did not significantly reduce neihter the coronary mortality (fatal MI) nor the morbidity (nonfatal MI). On the other hand, niacin (3 g/day) had a favorable effect on nonfatal MI, whereas it had not on coronary mortality [6].

Table II. Secondary prevention: lipid-lowering drugs

Reference	Drug	Results
3	estrogen 5 mg (1,119)	iatrogenic: (nonfatal MI)
4	dextrothyoxine 6 mg (1,110)	iatrogenic: ventricular premature contractions at entry (subgroup); fatal MI, nonfatal MI
5	estrogen 2.5 mg (1,101)	iatrogenic: thromboembolism, cancer mortality
6	clofibrate 1.8 mg (1,103)	fatal MI: n.s.; nonfatal MI: n.s.
6	niacin 3 g (1,119)	fatal MI: n.s.; nonfatal MI: significant reduction
15	clofibrate (497)	fatal MI: n.s.; SD, nonfatal MI ($p = 0.055$), total mortality: significant reduction
18	clofibrate (717)	baseline: angina → significant reduction in mortality, nonsignificant reduction in nonfatal MI baseline: MI → nonsignificant reduction in fatal and nonfatal MI
1	clofibrate + nicotinic acid (558)	total and CHD mortality: n.s.; nonfatal MI: significant reduction

Numbers in parentheses refer to the number of patients.

The Newcastle study [15] showed a significant reduction in total mortality and SD in subjects treated with clofibrate.

The Scottish study [18] showed positive results for patients with angina at entry, i. e., a significant reduction in total mortality in subjects treated with clofibrate. In a randomized controlled study using clofibrate plus niacin, *Carlson* et al. [1] observed a significant reduction in nonfatal MI but not in total CHD mortality.

In May 1980, the International Society and Federation of Cardiology convened the councils of Rehabilitation, Atherosclerosis and Epidemiology in Kronberg, FRG, in order to make a public policy report on secondary prevention [21].

On lipids, the panel stated: the controlled trial evidence justifying plasma lipid reduction in secondary prevention is very limited. Advice may be given on the following theoretical reasons: (1) hypercholesterolemia probably continues to aggravate CHD after MI, (2) to decrease progression of atherosclerosis and to support regression of existing arterial disease, (3) changes in dietary fat intake may diminish liability to thrombosis, and (4) to

Table III. Secondary prevention: smoking habits

Reference	Effect
22	62% reduction in mortality
14	significant independent discriminator for cardiac death
11	39% reduction in reinfarction
16	RR of cardiac death (S/ES: 2.7)
7	RR (S/NS) for coronary death or MI: 1.23
26	RR (S/Ex.S)for CV death or reinfarction: 2

No effect: *Weinblatt* et al. [25].

provide an education example to relatives of the patients. Personally, I would stress the importance of point 4.

What about cigarette smoking in secondary prevention? The CDP study [7] has shown, in the placebo group, an increase of about 25–30% for total mortality, cardiovascular mortality, SD, coronary mortality, nonfatal MI, and fatal and nonfatal MI in smokers as compared to nonsmokers. Several nonrandomized, but controlled studies have shown a significant decrease of between 30 and 50% in recurrent MI in subjects who stopped smoking soon after their MI [11, 13, 14, 16, 22, 26], but not all [25] (table III).

The Kronberg Group made the following statement: nonrandomized trials report a favorable effect of cessation of smoking (subsequent fatal MI or SD reduced by 20–30%). In fact, prevention is cheap, harmless, and much easier to achieve than in symptom-free subjects.

In the CDP study, a high systolic blood pressure was an independent risk factor for the recurrence of MI in the placebo group. To our knowledge, there are no controlled studies concerning the benefit of treatment of hypertension in MI subjects. The Kronberg Panel stated: treatment of hypertension should have a favorable influence on angina pectoris and on heart function.

In summary, the three main primary coronary risk factors high serum cholesterol, high blood pressure, and cigarette smoking are still predictors of recurrence of MI. The possible benefit of their modification does not rest on faultless randomized trials, but rather on indirect evidence. They should be tackled in a comprehensive rehabilitation program. Intervention during the whole of the rehabilitation program, by a qualified paramedical staff, should have a major impact on maintenance of life-style modification at least with regard to smoking.

References

1 Carlson, M. A.; Danielson, M.; Ekberg, I.; Klintemar, B.; Rosenhamer, B.: Reduction of myocardial reinfarction by the combined treatment with clofibrate and nicotinic acid. Atherosclerosis *28:* 81–86 (1977).

2 Coronary Drug Project Research Group: Factors influencing long-term prognosis after recovery from myocardial infarction. Three-year findings of the Coronary Drug Project, J. chron. Dis. *27:* 267–285 (1974).

3 Coronary Drug Project Research Group: Initial findings leading to modifications of its research protocol. J. Am. med. Ass. *214:* 1303–1313 (1970).

4 Coronary Drug Project Research Group: Findings leading to further modifications of its protocol with respect to dextrothyroxine. J. Am. med. Ass. *220:* 996–1008 (1972).

5 Coronary Drug Project Research Group: Findings leading to discontinuation of the 2.5 mg/day estrogen group. J. Am. med. Ass. *226:* 652–657 (1973).

6 Coronary Drug Project Research Group: Clofibrate and niacin in coronary heart disease. J. Am. med. Ass. *231:* 360–381 (1975).

7 Coronary Drug Project Research Group: Cigarette smoking as a risk factor in men with a prior history of myocardial infarction. J. chron. Dis. *32:* 415–425 (1979).

8 Kornitzer, M.; Denolin, H.: In Cachera, Bourassa, La maladie coronarienne, pp. 17–66 (Flammarion, Paris 1980).

9 Leren, P.: The effect of plasma cholesterol lowering diet in male survivors of myocardial infarction. A controlled trial. Acta med. scand., suppl. 466 (1966).

10 Marmorston, J.; Moore, F. J.; Hopkins, C. E.; Kuzma, O, T.; Weiner, J.: Clinical studies of long-term estrogen therapy in men with myocardial infarction. Proc. Soc. exp. Biol. Med. *110:* 400–408 (1962).

11 Matzdorff, F.; Lippert, A.; Schmidt, A.: Risiko-Indikatoren für den Reinfarkt. Dt. med. Wschr. *98:* 2183–2191 (1973).

12 Morrison, L. M.: Diet in coronary atherosclerosis, J. Am. med. Ass. *173:* 884–888 (1960).

13 Mulcahy, R.; Hickey, N.; Graham, I.; McKenzie, G.: Factors influencing longterm prognosis in male patients surviving a first coronary attack. Br. Heart J. *37:* 158–165 (1975).

14 Oxman, H. A.; Connolly, D. C.; Norbrega, L. R.: Factors influencing the subsequent prognosis of patients surviving their first myocardial infarction. Circulation 45: suppl. 2, p. 200 (1972).

15 Physicians of the Newcastle upon Tyne Region: Trial of clofibrate in the treatment of ischaemic heart disease. Five-year study. Br. med. J. *iv:* 767–775 (1971).

16 Pohjola, S.; Siltanen, P.; Romo, M.; Hwapakoski, J.: Effect of quitting smoking on the longterm survival after myocardial infarction. Proc, 2nd Scient. Meet. Working Group on Epidemiology and Prevention Eur. Soc. of Cardiology, No. 33 (1979).

17 Report of a Research Committee to the Medical Research Council.: Controlled trial of soya-bean oil in myocardial infarction. Lancet *ii:* 693–700 (1968).

18 Report by a Research Committee of the Scottish Society of Physicians: Ischaemic heart disease. A secondary prevention trial using clofibrate. Br. med. J. *iv:* 775–785 (1971).

19 Research Committee: Low-fat diet in myocardial infarction. A controlled trial. Lancet *ii:* 501–504 (1965).

20 Rose, G. A.; Thomson, W. B.; Williams, R. T. J.: Corn oil in treatment of ischaemic heart disease. Br. med. J. *i:* 1531–1533 (1965).
21 Secondary Prevention in Myocardial Infarction Survivors. J. Int. Soc. Fed. Cardiol., No. 3 (1980).
22 Sparrow, D.; Dawber, T. R.; Colton, T.: The influence of cigarette smoking on prognosis after a first myocardial infarction. J. chron. Dis. *31:* 425–432 (1978).
23 Stamler, J.; Pick, R.; Katz, L. N.; Pick, A.; Kaplan, B. M.; Berkson, D. M.; Century, D.: Effectiveness of estrogens for therapy of myocardial infarction in middle-age men. J. Am. med. Ass. *183:* 632–638 (1963).
24 Veterans Administration Cooperative Urological Research Group: Treatment and survival of patients with cancer of the prostate. Surgery Gynec. Obstet. *124:* 1011–1017 (1967).
25 Weinblatt, E.; Shapiro S.; Frank, Ch. W.; Sager, R. V.: Prognosis of men after first myocardial infarction. Mortality and first recurrence in relation to selected parameters. Am. J. publ. Hlth *58:* 1329–1347 (1968).
26 Wilhelmsson C.; Vedin, J. A.; Elmfeldt, D.; Tibblin, G.; Wilhelmsen, L.: Smoking and myocardial infarction. Lancet *i:* 415–420 (1975).

M. Kornitzer, MD, Université Libre de Bruxelles. Laboratoire d'Epidémiologie et de Médicine Sociale, route de Lennik, B–1070 Bruxelles (Belgium)

Adv. Cardiol., vol. 31, pp. 168–175 (Karger, Basel 1982)

Changes in Risk Factors among Participants in a Long-Term Exercise Rehabilitation Program

A. Oberman, P. Cleary, J. C. Larosa, H. K. Hellerstein, J. Naughton

Department of Preventive Medicine, The University of Alabama in Birmingham, Birmingham, Ala., USA

Introduction

Data from controlled randomized trials of exercise for patients after myocardial infarction (MI) support, though not definitively, the value of supervised exercise toward the secondary prevention of coronary heart disease [4]. These long-term benefits of physical activity for such patients may accrue through a variety of physiologic adaptations. One such mechanism postulated for the exercise program is the retardation of atherosclerosis by favorable attenuation of risk factors [6]. Moreover, it is universally accepted that individuals in physical activity programs will improve their sense of well-being, body image and generally adopt attitudes more conducive to a healthy life style.

At five participating clinical centers, the University of Alabama in Birmingham, Case Western Reserve University, Emory University, George Washington University and Lankenau Hospital, we have had the opportunity to study 651 men with a previous MI enrolled in a national collaborative trial of exercise for 3 years. The goals of the study were to determine the effects of medically prescribed and supervised physical activity on rehabilitation outcomes in men after MI. In this report we summarize the changes in smoking habits, blood pressure and lipids at 1 year for the control and exercise groups in the National Exercise and Heart Disease Project (NEHDP).

Methods

Candidates for the study had to be males 30–64 years old and to have had a documented acute MI within 3 years of admission. Participants were required to have a diastolic blood pressure (DBP) less than 100 mm Hg at supine rest, be able to exercise safely at a work load of at least 2 mph at a 3.5% grade on a treadmill and be without other impairments or coexisting disease likely to preclude long-term active participation. All patients first participated in a 6-week low-level physical activity program prior to randomization in order to acclimate them to the exercise program and test their willingness to return regularly to the exercise sessions. Those deemed eligible underwent evaluation before admission, and then semiannually during the study. Details of the study protocol have been described previously [5]. Risk factor assessment include smoking habits, alcohol intake, weight and a body fat index calculated as the sum of average skinfold readings at the triceps, subscapular and suprailiac areas. Resting blood pressure were taken with patients in the standing position. Fasting lipid measurements included total cholesterol, triglycerides, high-density lipoprotein cholesterol (HDL) and estimated low-density lipoprotein cholesterol (LDL) [3]. Complete lipid determinations were made only on a subset of 223 subjects enrolled in the George Washington and Case Western Reserve collaborating centers.

Intervention consisted solely of exercise training without any formal risk factor counseling. Patients with conditions requiring special attention were advised to seek medical counsel. The postrandomization exercise program was in two phases: (1) Patients exercised 3 days a week for the first 8 weeks at target levels on the basis of 85% of the maximal heart rate achieved on the baseline multistage exercise test (MSET). A 5-min warm-up and cool-down period was conducted before and after each session – 4 min on each of six stationary exercise devices with a 2-min rest period between the devices. (2) The long-term program consisted of supervised physical activities designed to yield the prescribed target heart rate. Activities included 15 min of continuous jogging, cycling or swimming followed by 25 min of games at three sessions per week.

Comparisons between exercise and control groups were made by t tests at baseline and analysis of covariance at 1 year. Using multiple regression techniques, 1-year means were adjusted for five independent variables: age, time from randomization, weight, work capacity at baseline, and the baseline value of the dependent variable.

Results

Description of Study Population

The participants were predominantly white, married, college-educated men with above-average incomes. Most (80%) had their qualifying MI more than 6 months before admission. The prevalence of smoking was 28%, history of hypertension 33%, elevated lipids 36% and a family history of coronary heart disease was reported in 31%. A high proportion, 85%, could not reach the 'age-predicted peak heart rate' on the admission MSET though 69% achieved a level of 7 METs or more. The exercise and

Table I. Percentage distribution of smoking habits at baseline and 1 year

Smoking habit	n	Baseline, % of total	n	1 year, % of baseline
Never				
Exercise	45	16.5	45	100.0
Control	45	16.9	44	97.9
Ex-smoker				
Exercise	148	54.2	120	81.1
Control	160	59.9	143	89.4
Current smoker				
Exercise	79	28.9	67	84.8
Control	62	23.2	58	93.6
Mean (SEM) n of cigarettes				
Exercise	54	18.0 (1.8)		19.2 (1.4)*
Control	45	19.1 (2.4)		21.6 (1.5)*

*Adjusted mean at 1 year.

control groups had similar baseline characteristics, the average ages were 52.0 and 51.5 years, respectively. After randomization, the exercise group increased work capacity from 7.9 to 8.3 METs and the control group decreased from 8.0 to 7.7 METs, a significant ($p < 0.0001$) difference at 1 year. This differential training effect occurred despite 'drop-outs' and 'drop-ins'. By the end of 1 year, approximately 6% of the exercise group continued exercising while 33% of the control group stated that they were exercising regularly.

Smoking

Neither overall smoking habits nor the amount of tobacco smoked were curtailed as a result of participating in the program (table I). Of those who had never smoked, 1 individual in the control group was noted to be smoking at 1 year. Ex-smokers in the exercise group tended to resume smoking more so than those in the control group: 19 versus 11%. The number of current smokers dropped by 15% in the exercise group and by 6% in the control group. Adjusted for baseline characteristics, the mean number of cigarettes smoked in both the exercise and control groups rose slightly. The few cigar and pipe smokers in the program did not change their smoking habits appreciably over the first year of the study. Among the 539 patients for whom we had classified smoking at 1 year, the change from baseline yielded a net gain in smoking of 5.5% for both groups.

Table II. Baseline and 1 year means of blood pressure (BP)

	n	Baseline mean (SEM)	1-year adjusted mean (SEM)
Systolic BP, mm Hg			
Exercise	273	125.0 (1.0)	125.8 (0.9)
Control	267	122.2 (1.0)	126.2 (0.9)
Diastolic BP, mm Hg			
Exercise	273	85.4 (0.6)	83.0 (0.5)
Control	267	84.4 (0.6)	84.4 (0.5)*

* $p < 0.03$.

Blood Pressure

To clarify the changes in blood pressure, it is important to consider several covariables – mainly obesity and alcohol intake. Body weight increased by 0.3 kg in the exercise group and by 1.2 kg in the controls (nonsignificant differences). In the exercise group the sum of the skinfolds decreased (50.5 to 48.5 mm), presumably representing a loss of body fat despite the slight weight gain, while the control group increased their skinfolds (49.4 to 50.8 mm) so that the group values at 1 year were different ($p < 0.05$). Alcohol consumption decreased from 6.3 to 5.9 oz per day for the exercise group whereas the controls showed a modest increment from 5.5 to 6.3 oz per day. Mean systolic blood pressure of the exercise group at baseline exceeded that of the controls ($p < 0.04$), however, the exercise group showed a lesser rise than the control group (table II). The adjusted means at 1 year were 125.8 and 126.2 mm Hg, respectively. The DBP were equivalent at baseline; the exercise group showed a 2.4-mm Hg decrease in contrast to an unchanged DBP in the control group so that at 1 year the adjusted means differed significantly ($p < 0.03$). This change in DBP may also be judged by the prevalence of hypertension (DBP > 95 mm Hg) over the 1-year period. There was a decline in the prevalence of hypertension from 17.0% at baseline to 12.1% at 12 months for the exercise group. The control group shows essentially the same trend but to a lesser extent, with baseline and 1-year values of 15.0 and 13.5%, respectively. Because of the possibility of confounding effects from drugs used for hypertension and angina, it is not possible to maintain a strictly controlled study for blood pressure. Other sources of bias in an exercise study include the more frequent visits of the exercise group and thus the greater likelihood of detecting and treating elevated blood pressure. However, in this study

Table III. Baseline and 1-year means of lipid measurements

	n	Baseline mean (SEM)	1-year adjusted mean (SEM)
Cholesterol, mg/dl			
Exercise	110	222.5 (3.3)	226.1 (2.3)
Control	113	220.2 (3.3)	231.3 (2.2)
LDL, mg/dl			
Exercise	108	150.1 (3.1)	153.1 (2.2)
Control	113	145.5 (3.1)	156.2 (2.2)
HDL, mg/dl			
Exercise	110	43.9 (1.0)	45.3 (0.9)
Control	113	44.4 (1.0)	44.7 (0.9)
Triglyceride, mg/dl			
Exercise	110	143.4 (5.8)	138.9 (5.5)*
Control	113	145.5 (7.1)	155.3 (5.4)*

*p < 0.04.

there were no significant differences in utilization of beta-blockers diuretics, antihypertensives or tranquilizers between exercise and control groups at 1 year.

Lipids

Only two of the five centers made complete lipid determinations. An analysis for those variables most likely to influence lipids demonstrated no significant 1-year change in body weight, alcohol consumption or smoking habits in this group of 223 patients. However, as with the larger group, the sum of skinfolds differed significantly ($p < 0.05$) between the exercise and control groups at 1 year. At 1 year, 73% of the exercise group were exercising while 31% of the control group reported engaging in regular exercise. Work capacity in this subset increased by 0.4 METs in the exercise group as contrasted to a decrease by 0,6 METs in the control group ($p < 0.0001$). Total cholesterol and LDL increased in both groups at 1 year but to a greater extent in the controls; HDL increased in both groups but slightly more in the exercise group, an increment of 1.4 mg/dl as opposed to 0.3 mg/dl in the controls (table III). Triglycerides in the exercise group dropped from 143.4 to 138.9 mg/dl while control group values increased from 145.5 to 155.3 mg/dl ($p < 0.04$).

Table IV. Summary of 1-year changes in risk factors and training variables in the exercise group

	1-year change		
	exercise	control	p value
Risk Factor			
Smoking cigarettes	±	±	n.s.
Blood pressure			
Systolic	+	++++	n.s.
Diastolic	−−−−	0	<0.03
Lipids			
Cholesterol	+	+++	n.s.
LDL	+	+++	n.s.
HDL	+	±	n.s.
Triglycerides	−	+	<0.04
Training variable			
Work capacity	++++	−−−−	<0.0001
Body fat	−−	++	<0.0005

+ (−) = Increase (decrease) of 1 SE from the mean at baseline to the 1-year adjusted mean.

Conclusion

In this randomized controlled study of supervised physical activity among male survivors of a prior MI, there were favorable trends in blood pressure and lipids but the magnitude of the changes do not appear to be of biologic importance. There was a net increase in smokers during the year after randomization. Despite some 'drop-outs' and 'drop-ins' between the control and exercise groups, work capacity improved differentially in the training group. Significant 1 year changes in the exercise group included: lower body fat, DBP, and triglycerides (table IV). Favorable trends also occurred in the exercise group as contrasted to the controls in total cholesterol, LDL and HDL.

These data do not dispel the notion that physical activity programs can substantially alter smoking habits, blood pressure and lipoprotein levels in different populations or at higher intensity levels of exercise. However, it is unlikely that 'coronary' patients in a supervised exercise program will exhibit marked improvement in major risk factors. This is not to say that a comprehensive rehabilitation program incorporating nutritional counseling and antismoking strategies might not be effective toward changing risk factors and long-term outcome [2]. Success in risk factor reduction might even be potentiated by an appropriate exercise program as suggested by the favorable trends noted in this controlled physical activity program.

It is also conceivable that the postulated benefits of exercise might accrue through modification of the influence of major risk factors without quantitative changes in the factors themselves. In the NEHDP, cigarette smokers in the exercise group were among those who extended their survival most as compared to their counterparts in the control group. Physical activity reduces heart rate and blood pressure at submaximal levels, alters carbon-monoxide metabolism [1], and decreases platelet aggregation [7]; any or all of these metabolic changes might counter the adverse effects of smoking. Nevertheless, until such mechanisms can be better delineated, it is unlikely that the benefits of exercise can be attributed to attenuation of smoking habits, blood pressure reduction or modification of lipids.

Acknowledgement

Collaborating investigators:

University of Alabama in Birmingham: *Albert Oberman,* MD, *Stephen Barton,* MD, *Glenda Barnes,* RN, *Del Eggert,* MEd; Case-Western Reserve University: *Herman K. Hellerstein,* MD, *Jorge Insua,* MD, *Chaim Yoran,* MD, *Paul Fardy,* PhD, *Barry A. Franklin,* PhD, *Krishna P. Kaimal,* MD; Emory University: *Charles Gilbert,* MD, *Daniel L. Blessing,* MD, *Barbara Johnson,* RN; George Washington University: *Patrick Gorman,* MD, *Margie LaVille,* RN, *Marcia Everett,* MS; Lankenau Hospital: *Alan Barry,* PhD, *James Daly,* MD, *John Satirsky,* MD, *William Marley,* PhD; Coordinating Centers: *Lawrence Shaw,* AM, *Paddy Cleary,* MS, *Jorge Rios,* MD, *Melvin Stern* MD, *Donald Paup,* PhD, *Dan Bogaty, Patti Kavanaugh, Sara Schlesselman,* MS, *John C. LaRosa,* MD, *John Naughton,* MD.

References

1 Cardiovascular disease, Sect. 4: Smoking and health: a report of the surgeon general, pp. 33–34. (US Department of Health, Education and Welfare, Public Health Service, 1979).

2 Kallio, V.; Hämäläinen, H.: Reduction in sudden deaths by a multifactorial intervention programme after acute myocardial infarction. Lancet *ii:* 1091–1094 (1979).

3 Lipid Research Clinical Manual of Laboratory Operations, vol. I. Lipid and lipoprotein analysis (DHEW, NIH Publication No. 75–628, 1974).

4 National Exercise and Heart Disease Project Staff: Effects of the prescribed supervised exercise program on mortality and cardiovascular morbidity in patients after a myocardial infarction. Am. J. Cardiol. *48:* 39–46 (1981).

5 Naughton, J.: The national exercise and heart disease project: development recruitment, and implementation; in Wenger, Exercise and the heart, pp. 205–222 (Cardiovas. Clin., Philadelphia 1978).

6 Oberman, A.; Kouchoukos, N. T.: Role of exercise after coronary artery bypass surgery; in Wenger, exercise and the heart, pp. 155–172 (Cardiovasc. Clin., Philadelphia 1978).

7 William, R. S,; Logue, E. E.; Lewis, J. L.; et al: Physical conditioning augments the fibrinolytic response to venous occlusion in healthy adults. New Engl. J. Med. *302:* 987–991 (1980).

A. Oberman, MD, Department of Preventive Medicine,
The University of Alabama in Birmingham, Birmingham, AL 35294 (USA)

Adv. Cardiol., vol. 31, pp. 176–179 (Karger, Basel 1982)

Risk Factor Modification in the Framework of Rehabilitation

Results of a Long-Term Rehabilitation Program in Bavaria

H. Angster, R. Glonner, M. Halhuber
Landesversicherungsanstalt Oberbayern, Munich, FRG

After an acute myocardial infarction (MI), 400 patients (blue-collar workers) of the Heart Hospital and Rehabilitation Center Höhenried near Munich (Bavarian National Health Insurance Co.), followed a comprehensive rehabilitation program for a period of 5 years (a twice yearly check-up after 6 weeks in the rehabilitation center) [1].

Methods

After discharge from the general hospital, the MI patient came as soon as possible to the rehabilitation center (generally after 2–4 weeks). During the 6 weeks of an early residential rehabilitation program, the patient underwent supervised physical training and was adjusted to the appropriate medication. Psychotherapy and health education was given in the frame of group sessions twice weekly. Psychologists and social workers were of assistance in solving psychosocial problems.

After leaving the rehabilitation center, all the 400 patients were under follow-up by two check-ups a year in the outpatients clinic of the Health Insurance Co.

In this paper only the long-term results concerning the risk factor modification are discussed, not the yearly mortality rate of 2.12% nor the return to work percentage (80% of the blue-collar workers).

Results

Table I shows the difference in the risk factor profile at the beginning of the rehabilitation program after the discharge from the general hospital (on admission to the Höhenried Rehabilitation Center), and the mean values after 8–10 follow-up examinations (twice yearly).

Table I. Risk factors present on admission (of inpatients) to Höhenried Rehabilitation Center and the mean values of 8–10 6-monthly follow-up examinations

	On admission to the center, %	Mean values of 8–10 follow-up examinations, %
Hypertension	23.3	5.8
Overweight (more than 10% overweight)	79.5 (50.0)	67.0 (34.9)
Cigarette smoking	69.5	25.3
Heavy smoking (15–30 cigarettes)	50.9	6.4
Hypercholesterolemia (over 280 mg%)	42.6	16.8
Hypertriglyceridemia	53.5	37.9
Hyperuricemia (8–12 mg%)	5.0	9.8

Figure 1 shows (in blood pressure, cholesterol, triglycerides) that a highly significant reduction of all known risk factors (except uric acid) took place during the patient's stay in the rehabilitation center and that during the follow-up period of 4–5 years, these values remained low.

Discussion

What are the conclusions of these observations?

(1) Early residential rehabilitation of MI patients in a specialized center is an efficient method to modify the classical risk factors and to change habits (e.g. the cessation of smoking as a secondary risk factor to change the prognosis) [2], even in lower social classes. The task of improving the personal life-style of the patient after MI needs special conditions of group psychotherapy and health education [3]. These conditions are more easily achieved in a specialized rehabilitation unit than in the traditional ward of a general hospital or in the office of the general physician. In Europe, we know of only one other study comparable to ours, concerning methods and sample (blue-collar workers), namely the Finnish study of *Kallio* et al. [4].

(2) Outpatients coronary group therapy and especially the follow-up examination (reevaluation) every 6 months seem to constitute a prolonged behavior therapy. Regular reexaminations are positive reinforcements for the patient. This open, but nonetheless organized supervised rehabilitation program, seems to us to be an effective way of improving the quality of life of the MI patient in the central European sociocultural setting.

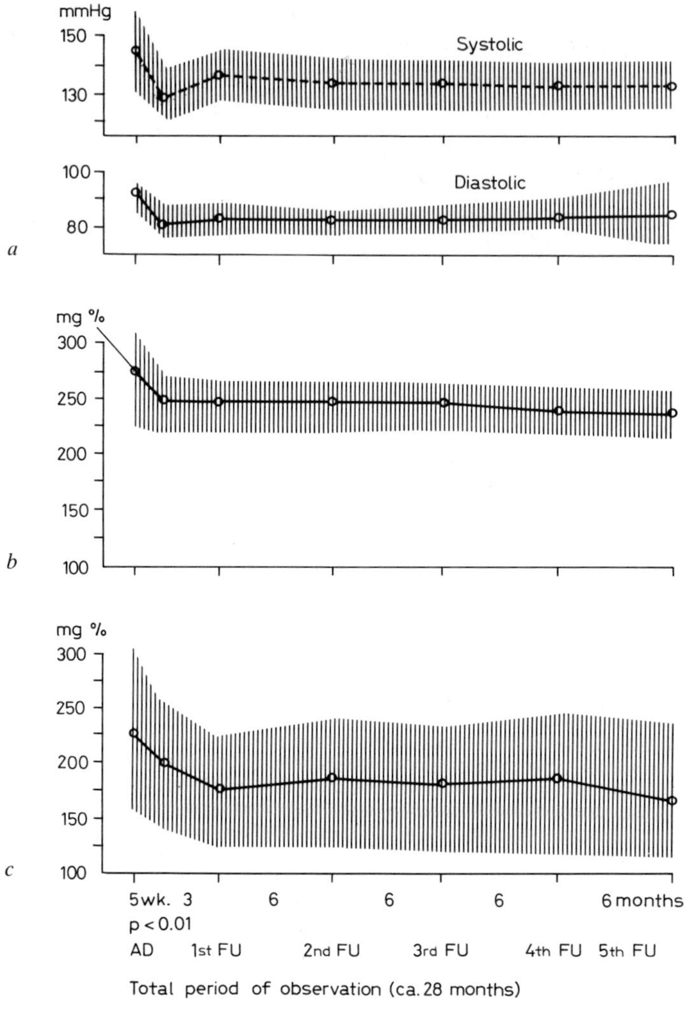

Fig. 1. Development of risk factors in MI patients of the Höhenried Rehabilitation Center. *a* Systolic and diastolic blood pressure (n = 293). *b* Levels of cholesterol (n = 293). *c* Levels of triglycerides (n = 282). A = admission; D = discharge; FU = follow-up.

References

1 Angster, H.; Glonner, R.: Medizinische und berufliche Rehabilitation Herzinfarktkranker durch umfassende Nachbetreuung (Ergebnisse der Beobachtung von 345 Herzinfarktpatienten über 6 Jahre)(LVA Oberbayern, München 1980).

2 Wilhelmsson, C.; Vedin, A.; Wilhelmsen, L.: Cost-benefit aspect of post-myocardial infarction intervention. Proc. Symp. on Acute and long-term management of myocardial ischemia, Oslo 1981. Acta med. scand., suppl. (1981).

3 Halhuber, M. J.: Health education in cardiac rehabilitation. Adv. Cardiol.,vol. 24, pp. 146–152 (Karger, Basel 1978).

4 Kallio, V.; Haemaelainen, H.; Hakkila, J.; Luurila, O.: Reduction of sudden death after a multifactorial intervention program in patients after acute myocardial infarction. Lancet Nov. 24, 1091 (1979).

M. J. Halhuber, MD, An der Gontardslust 17, D–5920 Bad Berleburg (FRG)

Adv. Cardiol., vol. 31, pp. 180–185 (Karger, Basel 1982)

Exercise and Health [1]

V. Froelicher

Cardiac Rehabilitation and Exercise Testing, School of Medicine,
University of California, University Hospital, San Diego, Calif., USA

Though many of us exercise and prescribe exercise for health reasons, there is no definitive evidence that this is effective in the prevention or reversal of coronary heart disease. The association between physical inactivity and the underlying atherosclerotic process is weak compared to other factors such as serum cholesterol, cigarette smoking, and hypertension. An inversely proportional association between the level of activity and degree of atherosclerosis has not been demonstrated. Physical inactivity does not necessarily precede the atherosclerotic process and epidemiological studies have been performed without finding physical inactivity as a risk factor. Often physical inactivity was not found to be an independent risk factor since other risk factors and markers concentrated in the inactive group. The capacity of physical inactivity to predict coronary events has not been reproducible when applied to different populations nor has the exercise hypothesis been documented by autopsy studies.

Epidemiologists have had difficulty documenting the health benefits of exercise because of numerous problems including: selection and premorbid job transfers; quantifying activity levels; accurate diagnosis of coronary disease; and variability of risk prediction in different populations. In addition, the type of exercise that is beneficial and its method of protection is uncertain. The beneficial action may be mediated by hormonal and clotting factor changes as shown by the exercise-induced lowering of catecholamine levels and increase in fibrinolysis. Recent studies continue to have limitations, but *Paffenbarger* et al. [1, 2] and *Morris* et al. [3] have found physical inactivity to be a risk factor in three different apparently well

[1] Supported by Specialized Center of Research on Ischemic Heart Disease, NIH Research grant HL 17682 awarded by the National Heart, Lung and Blood Institute to *John Ross,* MD.

populations and provide some quantification of protective activity levels. Fortunately, high levels of activity (i.e., marathoning) are not necessary and modest levels of exercise provide a decreased probability of developing coronary disease.

Echocardiography has been utilized to evaluate cardiac adaptations to exercise training in longitudinal studies [4]. Reported cardiac changes secondary to endurance training in young subjects have included increased ventricular mass, wall thickness, and volume. However, echocardiographic measurements of other groups of young subjects and older subjects failed to document these changes in spite of improvement in maximal oxygen consumption. Our study in coronary patients found no change in myocardial mass after 6 months of cardiac rehabilitation [5]. These echocardiographic studies suggest that increases in left ventricular mass may not occur in younger subjects unless higher levels of training are used and may never occur in older subjects, particularly those with coronary disease.

Animal studies have provided substantial evidence of the cardiovascular benefits of regular physical activity. Improved coronary circulation has been demonstrated in exercise trained animals by increased coronary artery size, capillary density, reduced myocardial infarction size, and maintenance of coronary flow in response to hypoxia. However, the data on changes in collateral perfusion is controversial [6, 7]. Studies utilizing various animal models have reported improvement in cardiac function secondary to exercise training. Improved intrinsic contractility, faster relaxation, enzymatic alterations, calcium availability and enhanced autonomic and hormonal control of function have all been implicated. The primate study by *Kramsch* et al. [8] demonstrated beneficial changes and lessening of atherosclerotic lesions which is most encouraging. This is the most important animal study supporting the use of exercise in the primary prevention of atherosclerosis. There have been few other animal studies of primary prevention, most dealing with the indirect effect of exercise on blood pressure and lipids and they have not provided support for the exercise hypothesis [4, 6].

Exercise training can be effective in achieving the physiological, psychological, and vocational goals of cardiac rehabilitation [9]. However, two recent randomized trials of the effect on morbidity and mortality have found no difference between controls and exercised post-myocardial infarction patients [10, 11]. Perhaps the greatest benefits of exercise are an increase in the anginal threshold and in functional capacity which could be due to noncardiac adaptations. Changes in cardiac function and coronary blood flow secondary to exercise in man remain unproven and it is unlikely that exercise has a direct effect on the atherosclerotic process. The beneficial changes in hemodynamic measurements and work capacity secondary to an exercise program in patients with coronary disease could be due to changes in the peripheral circulation, the sympathetic nervous systems, catecholamine levels, and skeletal muscles rather than cardiac alterations. Hemodynamic and work capacity changes that occur within several months of training in older subjects are most likely due to noncardiac peripheral changes and longer periods of training are needed for cardiac alterations [12]. If cardiac alterations could be demonstrated and if either improvement or worsening could be identified, the physician could feel more secure in his recommendation for or against exercise for his coronary patient.

Perfext is a randomized study of the effects of supervised exercise on myocardial perfusion and function conducted by the Cardiac Rehabilitation and Exercise Testing Program at the University of California, San Diego Medical Center. Perfext is an acronym for *per*formance, *per*fusion, *ex*ercise *tr*ial. The study is being supported by the National Institutes of Health in order to scientifically evaluate exercise programs for cardiac patients using new nuclear cardiac imaging techniques.

During an initial 3-year pilot period, we found improvements in heart function and perfusion after 6 months of an exercise program, possibly due to exercise in selected patients [13, 14]. Nuclear scanning of the patients showed improved blood flow to the heart and improved heart function in some of the first patients. After these preliminary findings, a randomized trial was initiated. 1 year between radionuclide exercise tests is planned for both the exercisers and the controls.

Men between the ages of 35 and 65 who have stable coronary artery disease are considered candidates for Perfext. They must have one or more of the following: previous heart attack, coronary artery disease, angina pectoris or coronary artery bypass surgery.

Patients undergo a thallium treadmill test and a supine bicycle ventriculogram to evaluate blood flow to heart muscle and heart function during exertion. These tests are free and the results are sent to the referring physician. On completion of the initial tests, a computerized coin-flip assigns the patient to an exercise group or a control group. Patients in the exercise group participate in a year of medically supervised exercise training. Patients in the control group are assigned to usual care, including instructions for a walking program. The tests are repeated after 1

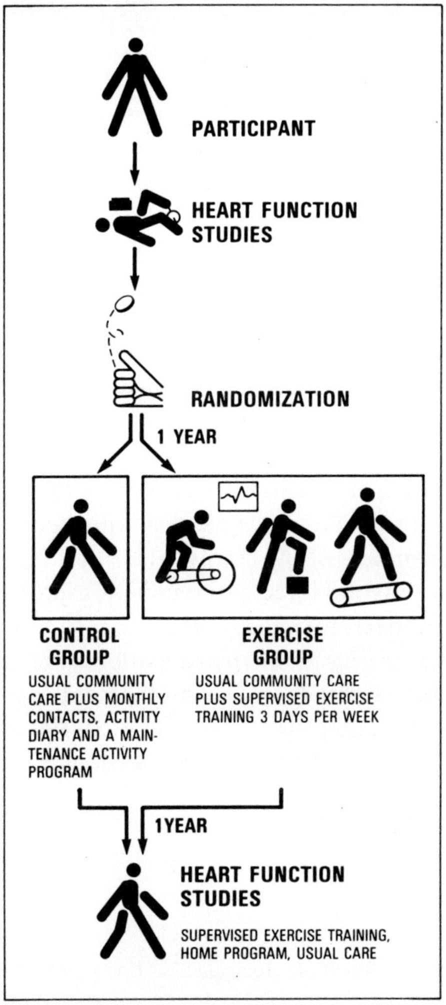

Fig. 1. Protocol for Perfext, a randomized study of the effects of exercise on the hearts of patients with coronary heart disease. The heart function studies used are radionuclide exercise tests of both function and perfusion. This study, sponsored by the NHLBI at UCSD is at no cost to accepted patients.

year. Control patients are then offered the medically supervised exercise program. The study is illustrated in figure 1. Both groups can attend a series of educational classes which give information on diet, stress, and risk factors.

Patients need not refrain from taking any medications during the Perfext study. However, there is a gradual tapering of beta-blockers and digoxin prior to radionuclide exercise testing. Only after physician approval with reassurance that this can be done safely will the patient be allowed to participate in Perfext.

The physician may be apprehensive about losing a patient or relinquishing control of a patient entered into such a clinical trial. However, patients participating in research trials remain under the care of their primary physician, and are referred for management to their own physician for new medical problems arising or detected during the clinical trials. Randomized trials like Perfext are designed to provide the clinician with answers to dilemmas encountered daily in clinical practice.

Because the pattern of care is based on information derived from previous patients with the same medical problem, patients and physicians should understand the value of clinical research trials such as Perfext. A patient's participation in a clinical trial augments medical knowledge thus helping the individual patient, members of his family, and other patients. The referring physician serves as a pivotal force in this complex interaction – critically assessing the proposed trial, selecting patients appropriate for entry and counselling them regarding their participation. Academic reseachers are anxious for this opportunity to work with their colleagues in practice and would do nothing to undermine a patient's confidence or lessen the patient's sense of well-being derived from the doctor-patient relationship.

References

1 Paffenbarger, R. S.; Brand, R. J.; Sholtx, R. I.; Jung, D. L.: Energy expenditure, cigarette smoking, and blood pressure level as related to death from specific diseases. Am. J. Epidem. *108:* 12 (1978).

2 Paffenbarger, R. S.; Wing, A. L.; Hyde, R. T.: Physical activity as an index of heart attack risk in college alumni. Am. J. Epidem. *108:* 161 (1978).

3 Morris, J. N.; Pollard, R.; Everitt, M. G.; Chave, S. P. W.; Semmence, A. M.: Vigorous exercise in leisure time: protection against coronary heart disease. Lancet *ii:* 1207 (1980).

4 Froelicher V. F.: Exercise testing and training (LeJacq Publishers, New York 1982).

5 Ditchey, R. V.; Watkins, J.; McKirnan, M. D.; Froelicher, V. F.: Effects of exercise training on left ventricular mass in patients with ischemic heart disease. Am. Heart J. *101:* 701 (1981).

6 Froelicher, V. F.; Brown, P.: Exercise and coronary heart disease. J. Card. Rehab. *4:* 277 (1981).

7 Sanders, M.; White, F. C.; Peterson, T. M.; Bloor, C. M.: Effects of endurance exercise on coronary collateral blood flow in miniature swine. Am. J. Physicol. *234:* H614 (1978).
8 Kramsch, D. M.; Aspen, A. J.; Abramowitz, B. M.; Abell, M. A.; Hood, W. B.: Cardiovascular effects of exercise in primate atherosclerosis. Circulation *59/60:* 652 (1979).
9 Wilson, P.; Fardy, P.; Froelicher, V.: Cardiac rehabilitation, adult fitness, and exercise testing (Lea & Febiger, Philadelphia 1981).
10 Shaw, L. W.: Effects of a prescribed supervised exercise program on mortality and cardiovascular morbidity in myocardial infarction subjects. Am. J. Cardiol. *48:* 39 (1981).
11 Rechnitzer P. A.: The effect of exercise prescription on the recurrence rate of myocardial infarction in men (Abstract). Am. J. Cardiol. *47:* 419 (1981).
12 Paterson, D. H.; Shephard, R. J.; Cunningham, D.; Jones, N. L.; Andrew, G.: Effects of physical training on cardiovascular function following myocardial infarction. J. appl. Physiol. *47:* 482 (1979).
13 Froelicher, V. F.; Jensen, D. G.; Atwood, E.; McKirnan, M. D.; Gerber, K.; Slutsky, R.; Battler, A.; Ashburn, W.; Ross, J., Jr.: Cardiac rehabilitation: evidence for improvement in myocardial perfusion and function. Archs phys. Med. Rehabil. *61:* 517 (1980).
14 Jensen, D.; Atwood, J. E.; Froelicher, V.; McKirnan, M. D.; Battler, A.; Ashburn, W.; Ross, J., Jr.: Improvement in ventricular function during exercise studied with radionuclide ventriculography after cardiac rehabilitation. Am. J. Cardiol. *46:* 770 (1980).

V. Froelicher, MD, Associate Professor of Medicine, Cardiac Rehabilitation and Exercise Testing, School of Medicine, University of California, University Hospital, 225 Dickinson Street, San Diego, CA 92103 (USA)

Adv. Cardiol., vol. 31, pp. 186–190 (Karger, Basel 1982)

Rationale of Physical Training in Patients with Angina pectoris

Robert A. Bruce, Kenneth F. Hossack

Department of Medicine, Division of Cardiology, RG-20,
University Hospital, Seattle, Wash., USA

Introduction

Patients with angina pectoris typically experience transient chest discomfort or pain with exertion or emotion which is relieved by rest and/or nitroglycerin. In most instances it is due to significant stenosis of coronary arteries due to atherosclerosis. In some patients other causes, such as 'tight' aortic stenosis and marked left ventricular hypertrophy without arterial disease, may manifest angina whenever hemodynamic load initiates a myocardial demand for oxygenated blood that substantially exceeds a virtually normal supply of coronary blood flow. Thus angina is a syndrome which may occur from a variety of causes. When patients with coronary disease become symptomatic exercise capacity is limited, physical deconditioning ensues, and risks of cardiac events or complications increase. Physical exercise increases the heart rate, systolic pressure, pressure-rate product, subendocardial wall tension and stress, and therefore myocardial oxygen requirements. Accordingly, it seems paradoxical that physical training is either indicated or should be beneficial in such patients. Yet the primary objectives of such training are to enhance peripheral adaptive mechanisms which increase the functional aerobic capacity and reverse the physical deconditioning imposed by chronic disease. The secondary objectives are the associated minor increase in arterial oxygen supply, diminished relative aerobic requirements and cardiac responses of submaximal exertion which spare the ischemic and/or infarcted heart.

Methods

Standardized multistage exercise tests [4] of symptom-limited exercise are necessary to define the severity of cardiac impairment before initiating training. Testing should be repeated in about 2–3 months to determine objectively whether beneficial physiologic adaptations have been achieved; if not, patients often need other studies to ascertain the feasibility of coronary bypass surgery.

Training should involve dynamic, endurance and interval types of exercise of several muscle groups, in an appropriately supervised and monitored environment with emergency treatment facilities available. It should last for thirty minutes and be repeated about 3 times weekly for several weeks. Use of nitroglycerin just before exercise conditioning provides some acute prophylactic benefits because of a reduction in submaximal blood pressure and an increase in maximal oxygen uptake [5] which facilitates training provided blood pressure does not drop below the usual levels.

Results

Numerous studies indicate that physiologic adaptations occur after several weeks of training [7]. These include (1) increased functional aerobic capacity or maximal oxygen uptake due to increased arterial oxygen content and arterial mixed venous oxygen difference; (2) no change in absolute amount of weight-adjusted oxygen requirements at rest or during the same activities which correspond to submaximal workloads. (3) Since the numerator of absolute oxygen cost for the same physical activity remains constant, but the denominator of maximal oxygen uptake or aerobic capacity increases, the ratio, or relative aerobic cost of submaximal exertion is lowered somewhat. Inasmuch as cardiac responses to metabolic needs are scaled to the *relative aerobic requirement,* rather than to the absolute level, heart rate, cardiac output, systolic pressure, pressure-rate product and subendocardial wall tension are proportionately reduced [7]. This reduction in demand, therefore, represents a secondary benefit of exercise conditioning which effectively spares the ischemic and/or infarcted heart. Additionally, a minor increase in arterial oxygen content enhances supply and permits greater peripheral extraction, or widened arterial-mixed venous oxygen difference. Accordingly, ECG evidence of ischemic ST depression, at submaximal exertion, which reflects *changes in the balance* of supply of oxygenated blood and hemodynamic demand, is lessened [6]. Often chest discomfort or pain, as subjective manifestations of ischemia, is also diminished or eliminated.

Adherence to physical training programs in a community organization that is appropriately supervised provides additional psychosocial benefits of shared experiences and improves strategies for coping with life stresses. Unfortunately, cumulative nonadherence, either because of progression of cardiovascular disease or other socioeconomic factors becomes a problem [1].

Even if adherence is well maintained for 2 years, invasive studies show evidence of continuing peripheral adaptation with further increments in arterial oxygen content and A–$\overline{V}$ oxygen difference [3]. Heart rate and pulmonary arterial pressure during moderate exercise may be lower. For the majority of patients who do not maintain a high maximal oxygen uptake, despite the same peripheral responses, further cardiac impairment is manifested by a lower stroke volume and cardiac output at the same levels of energy expenditure. Indeed, the peripheral adaptations may obscure or postpone clinical manifestations of progression of coronary heart disease. Whereas serial measurements of maximal oxygen uptake may identify these patients, invasive studies with catheterization of pulmonary and systemic arteries are necessary to reveal the cardiac mechanisms involved.

Two cases are cited to illustrate the broad spectrum of clinical disease and its management.

(1) WB, a 54-year-old, obese (116 kg) man was admitted with preinfarction angina, agitated depression, denial and evolved an extensive anterior myocardial infarction and cardiomegaly. With medical management he stabilized, had very low exercise tolerance at discharge due to hypotension, (consistent with a very high mortality risk) yet gradually became more active, lost weight and accepted psychotherapy. Because of symptoms and limitations, coronary arteriography was performed at 6 weeks and showed extensive disease, but he refused bypass surgery. With continued activity, unsupervised, he showed substantial clinical and physiologic improvement by 10 weeks which has been maintained for nearly 1 year.

(2) RMcA, a 68-year-old, hypertensive diabetic with angina entered and continued with a supervised physical training program for 5 years. He then developed atrial fibrillation, revealed exertional left ventricular dysfunction, and had bypass grafting of 4 severely diseased coronary arteries. At 74 he resumed physical training, further increased his aerobic and cardiac capacities, and became very active in community affairs.

The role of propranolol, a beta-blocker, in relation to exercise testing and training, warrants two comments. Heart rate is slower, blood pressure and mixed venous oxygen content are lower and A-$\overline{V}$ oxygen difference is wider, but effects on maximal cardiac output and oxygen uptake vary inversely with severity of cardiac functional impairments [2]. Often patients are taking a beta-blocker while participating in physical training. Then the prescription for heart rate limits is altered in actual beats per minute, but not if rates are prescribed at the same percentages of the reduced maximal heart rate during beta blockade [8].

Finally, it should be emphasized that heart rate and cardiac output at maximal exercise are more likely to be increased by bypass surgical grafting to revascularize the myocardium [10] than by physical conditioning.

Discussion and Conclusions

Appropriately supervised exercise training programs can be effective in patients with angina pectoris due to ischemic or coronary heart disease. Continued training is necessary to maintain the peripheral adaptations which *secondarily* spare the ischemic and/or infarcted heart. If the threshold for angina is raised and patients exceed 85% of their maximal heart rate, they may become vulnerable to cardiac arrest. Other factors also contribute to this relatively rare risk. Fortunately, with prompt defibrillation of the ventricles, virtually all may be converted to normal sinus rhythm without significant sequelae. Even with clinical benefit and no recurrence of exertional symptoms many patients may develop further cardiac impairment. Failure to maintain an adequate age-adjusted maximal oxygen uptake may be an important clue to detection of this phenomenon [9]. Sooner or later, these patients are likely to need definitive diagnostic studies to ascertain severity of coronary arterial disease and feasibility of coronary bypass surgery. Such patients may then attain higher heart rates, cardiac output and oxygen uptake at maximal exertion [10]. Maximal clinical benefit is achieved when physical training is resumed to acquire and maintain the additional peripheral adaptive benefits.

References

1 Bruce, E. H.; Frederick, R,; Bruce, R. A.; Fisher, L. D.: Comparison of active participants and dropouts in CAPRI cardiopulmonary rehabilitation programs. Am. J. Cardiol. *37:* 53–60 (1976).

2 Bruce, R. A.; Hossack, K. F.; Kusumi, F.; Clarke, J. L.: Acute effects of oral propranolol on hemodynamic responses to upright exercise. Am. J. Cardiol. 44: 132–140 (1979).

3 Bruce, R. A.; Kusumi, F.; Frederick, R.: Differences in cardiac function with prolonged physical training for cardiac rehabilitation. Am. J. Cardiol. *40:* 597–603 (1977).

4 Bruce, R. A.; Kusumi, F.; Hosmer, D.: Maximal oxygen intake and nomographic assessment of functional aerobic impairment in cardiovascular disease. Am. Heart J. *85:* 546–562 (1973).

5 Detry, J-M. R.; Bruce, R. A.: Effects of nitroglycerin on 'maximal' oxygen intake and exercise electrocardiogram in coronary heart disease. Circulation *43:* 155–163 (1971).
6 Detry, J. M.; Bruce, R. A.: Effects of physical training on exertional S-T segment depression in coronary heart disease. Circulation *44:* 390–396 (1971).
7 Detry, J-M. R.; Rousseau, M.; Vandenbroucke, G.; Brasseur, L.; Kusumi, F.; Bruce, R. A.: Increased arteriovenous oxygen difference after physical training in coronary heart disease. Circulation *44:* 109–118 (1971).
8 Hossack, K. F.; Bruce, R. A.; Clarke, L. J.: Influence of propranolol on exercise prescription of training heart rates. Cardiology *65:* 47–58 (1980).
9 Hossack, K. F.; Bruce, R. A.; Green, B,; Kusumi, F.; DeRouen, T. A.; Trimble, S.: Maximal cardiac output during upright exercise: approximate normal standards and variations with coronary heart disease. Am. J. Cardiol *46:* 204–212 (1980).
10 Hossack, K. F.; Bruce, R. A.; Kusumi, F.; Ritterman, J.; Ivey, T. D.; Bailey, W. B.: Increased maximal cardiac output following bypass surgery (Abstract). Aust. N. Z. J. Med. *11:* 471–472 (1981).

R. A. Bruce, MD, Department of Medicine, Division of Cardiology, RG-20, University Hospital, Seattle, WA 98195 (USA)

Adv. Cardiol., vol. 31, pp. 191–198 (Karger, Basel 1982)

Exercise Therapy in Patients with Angina pectoris

Roy J. Shephard

School of Physical and Health Education, Department of Preventive Medicine and Biostatistics, and Institute of Medical Sciences, University of Toronto, and Toronto Rehabilitation Centre, Toronto, Ont., Canada

Prognosis in Angina

Angina – particularly angina of effort – has a poor prognosis in the absence of effective treatment. *Hughes* et al. [13] observed a 2-year mortality of 15.7% in severely affected patients who were receiving anticoagulants; 27.5% of their sample developed a clinical myocardial infarct over the same period. More recently, a 10% mortality over 3 years was reported for patients with chronic stable angina, whether treated by medical or surgical means [24].

Given this gloomy outlook, it is hardly surprising there has been interest in the value of exercise therapy [17, 19, 33]. This brief article will examine the rationale for exercise treatment of angina pectoris.

Value of Exercise Therapy

Most authors have found an exercise programme to be helpful in angina pectoris. *Kattus* [14] noted that three quarters of anginal patients showed an improved treadmill exercise tolerance following participation in a daily walking programme. *Redwood* et al. [26] commented on a consistent improvement of exercise tolerance as a result of physical training. Our laboratory has observed a substantial gain of oxygen transport in response to an interval training regimen [16], and in 96 of 192 patients angina was no longer a feature of exercise testing after 3 years of postcoronary rehabilitation [15].

Nevertheless, there is some danger that excessive activity may provoke acute cardiac failure in the patient with severe myocardial ischaemia [25], and a high proportion of fatalities in postcoronary rehabilitation programmes are found among patients with angina and/or deep ST segmental depression [28]. Moreover, patients with ST segmental depression are particularly prone to die during periods of physical activity [28], although there is no evidence that their overall prospects are worsened by exercise training [15].

Mechanisms for Relief of Anginal Pain

The symptom of angina arises from a mismatching of myocardial oxygen consumption and oxygen delivery to the cardiac muscle. As a result of the mismatch, anaerobic metabolites accumulate in sufficient quantities to cause symptoms ranging from discomfort to severe pain. At least five tactics could theoretically relieve symptoms: (i) an increase of pain threshold; (ii) an increase of coronary blood flow; (iii) a redistribution of coronary blood flow; (iv) an increase of myocardial oxygen extraction, and (v) a decrease of cardiac energy expenditure.

Increase of Pain Threshold

Patients vary widely in their pain threshold. Some individuals show deep ST depression with no complaints, while others have severe pain despite little electrocardiographic change.

It is very likely that psychological factors raise the pain threshold with many types of treatment, exercise included. *Bergman and Varnauskas* [3] demonstrated a reduction of symptoms in response to placebo tablets, while *Zohman and Tobis* [36] noted a placebo effect from the breathing of compressed air. *Kellermann* et al. [18] compared homeopathic calisthenics with a dose of ergometer training that was sufficient to augment oxygen transport capacity. Although the course of homeopathic exercise was physiologically ineffective, it nevertheless enabled patients to exercise to a significantly higher heart rate before the onset of anginal pain.

Increase of Coronary Blood Flow

(1) Vascular changes. Animal experiments suggest that training can (a) enlarge the basic dimensions of the coronary vascular tree [31], and (b)

facilitate blood flow to ischaemic regions of the myocardium by opening up collateral branches [8]. Unfortunately, the normal human subject reaches close to maximal coronary vasodilatation in all-out exercise [32], and there is little reason to suppose that any mechanism could augment flow in the rigid, sclerosed vessels of a typical anginal patient. Certainly, attempts to demonstrate a stimulation of collateral formation by exercise in human ischaemic heart disease have to date been unconvincing [9, 35].

Changes of Wall Tension. Flow to most of the left ventricle is occluded throughout the systolic phase of the cardiac cycle, because intramural tension exceeds the perfusing pressure at the coronary ostia [12]. The relationship between intraventricular pressure P and wall tension T is described by the Laplace relationship:

$$T = P/h\ (R_1R_2/R_1+R_2),$$

where R_1 and R_2 are the principal radii of the heart and h is the wall thickness [22].

The intramural pressure is thus decreased, relative to perfusing pressure, if the end-diastolic volume is diminished. The influence of training upon cardiac dimensions is complex. Cardiac hypertrophy and an increase of blood volume tend to augment the end-diastolic volume, but an increase of myocardial contractility has the opposite effect. The net result is often little change of the Laplace relationship. However, if cardiac hypertrophy occurs, tension is distributed over a larger cross-section of muscle and can be opposed by the development of a lesser force within individual myofibrils. Vigorous and sustained training produces substantial hypertrophy in a young healthy heart, but it is unlikely that a severely disabled anginal patient can achieve a sufficient intensity of training to achieve such a result.

Changes of Cycle Length. A third important mechanism improving coronary flow is a decrease of exercise heart rate. Coronary perfusion is largely a diastolic phenomenon, and unfortunately tachycardia develops almost entirely at the expense of the diastolic phase of the cardiac cycle. Thus, if training reduces the heart rate at a given workload, the coronary flow will automatically be improved.

Redistribution of Coronary Flow

Even if total coronary flow remains unchanged after physical training, it is conceivable that a redistribution of the available blood flow may occur. Normally, the most poorly perfused tissue lies in the immediate subendocardial zone. Much of the coronary flow is directed to more superficial tissues ('proximal steal') [21]. A decrease of intramural tension could help to redress this balance, allowing a relative improvement of subendocardial perfusion. Reflex narrowing of the proximal branches or a dilatation of alternative deep pathways could have similar effects.

Increase of Myocardial Oxygen Extraction

There is some evidence that training increases the myocardial oxygen extraction, at least marginally [34]. One potential mechanism for a widened coronary arteriovenous oxygen difference is an increase of hemoglobin level, and thus of arterial oxygen content. A second possibility is a shift of the oxygen dissociation curve, brought about either by changes in red cell 2:3-diphosphoglycerate or an alteration of local pH. Finally, a few authors have hinted that training may increase myocardial enzyme activity [1]; however, even if this minority opinion is substantiated, it has yet to be demonstrated that enzyme concentrations play a significant role in limiting myocardial oxygen utilization.

Decrease of Cardiac Energy Expenditure

There is little scope for reducing the energy expenditures associated with the basal metabolism of the heart, electrochemical reactions, or the internal work of fibre shortening. Attention must thus be directed to the two principal components of cardiac work – the internal energy expenditure needed to develop intramural tension, and the useful external work performed in pumping the stroke volume against arterial pressure.

Decrease of Heart Rate. The total workload of the heart is approximated by the pulse-pressure product, given relatively constant cardiac dimensions. A decrease of heart rate at any given power output thus reduces the cardiac cost of the activity [19, 20, 29].

Decrease of Blood Pressure. Habituation, a lesser output of catecholamines, a strengthening of the skeletal muscles, and a lessening of central and peripheral drive may all cause some reduction of blood pressure and thus tension work following training [7].

Decrease of Cardiac Output. The cardiac output required for a given power output may be decreased by an improvement of mechanical efficiency. Tasks such as uphill treadmill running and cycle ergometry are unfamiliar to older patients, so that efficiency improves 5–10% with repetition of the test [30]. It has also been argued that an increase of skeletal muscle enzyme concentrations may allow a wider systemic arteriovenous oxygen difference and a lower muscle blood flow during submaximal work [4].

Changes of Myocardial Contractility. Training usually increases myocardial contractility, augmenting myocardial oxygen consumption. As in skeletal muscle, the useful component of cardiac work (pressure/volume work) depends markedly upon the velocity of muscle contraction. The rate of shortening is influenced somewhat by external loading and the properties of the series elastic elements, but the main determinant of contraction velocity and thus the amount of external work performed by the heart is myocardial contractility.

At heavy loads, as during exercise, a slow contraction improves efficiency. However, in vivo, the disadvantages of a training-induced speeding of contraction may be offset by other factors, including a reduction of ventricular size and a decreased output of catecholamines at any given work rate. Overall changes of left ventricular function are generally minimal when anginal patients are investigated before and after training [2, 6].

When first seen, many patients with anginal symptoms have a poor myocardial contractility, with a stiffening of the ventricular wall [9, 11]. If activity is pursued too vigorously in the face of anginal pain, a vicious cycle of diminishing stroke volume, increasing end-diastolic volume, increased tension work and cardiac failure may be established [23, 25]. Beta-blocking drugs reduce the positive inotropic and chronotropic response to exercise, and possibly have some negative inotropic effect in their own right [10]. The resultant decrease of heart rate, wall stress and contractility may reduce myocardial oxygen consumption and thus help the patient with angina. However, if the patient is already close to cardiac failure, the combination of exercise and beta-blocking drugs may induce the vicious cycle already discussed [27]. Likewise, in some patients digitalis may help exercise tolerance, the direct costs of increased myocardial contractility being more than offset by a decrease of heart size and wall stress [5].

Conclusions

Training can do little to reopen stenosed vessels, and the main rationale for any exercise programme is to enable a patient to develop a greater power output for the same pressure-rate product. Nevertheless, small increases of the limiting double-product may result from increased pain tolerance, increased general and local myocardial perfusion and increased oxygen extraction. The avenues of benefit are such that as many as 50% of anginal patients can be helped greatly by a regular programme of endurance exercise.

References

1 Barnard, R. J.: Long-term effects of exercise on cardiac function. Exercise Sports Sci. Rev. *3:* 113–133 (1975).

2 Battler, A.; Froelicher, V.; Slutsky, R.; McKirnan, D.; Strong, M. L.; Ashburn, W.; Ross, J.: Initial observations of changes in ventricular function after exercise in coronary disease patients. Circulation *59/60 (II):* 21 (1979).

3 Bergman, H.; Varnauskas, E.: Placebo effect in physical training of coronary heart disease; in Larsen, Malmborg, Coronary heart disease and physical fitness (Munksgaard, Copenhagen 1971).

4 Clausen, J. P.: Circulatory adjustment to dynamic exercise and effect of physical training in normal subjects and in patients with coronary artery disease. Prog. cardiovasc. Dis. *18:* 459–495 (1976).

5 Covell, J. W.; Braunwald, E.; Ross, J.; Sonnenblick, E. H.: Studies on digitalis XVI. Effects on myocardial oxygen consumption. J. clin. Invest. *45:* 1535–1542 (1966).

6 Detry, J. M.; Rousseau, R. L.; Vandenbroucke, M.; Kusumi, F.; Brasseur, L. A.; Bruce, R. A.: Increased arteriovenous oxygen difference after physical training in coronary disease. Circulation *44:* 109–118 (1971).

7 Dressendorfer R. H.; Amsterdam, E. A.; Mason, D. T.: Therapeutic effects of exercise training in angina patients; in Cohen, Mock, Ringqvist, Physical conditioning and cardiovascular rehabilitation, pp. 121–138 (Wiley, New York 1981).

8 Eckstein, R.: Effect of exercise and coronary artery narrowing on coronary collateral circulation. Circulation Res. *5:* 230–235 (1957).

9 Ellerstad, M. H.: Stress testing. Principles and practice (Davis, Philadelphia 1975).

10 Epstein, S. E.; Braunwald, E.: Beta-adrenergic receptor blocking drugs. New Engl. J. Med. *275:* 1106–1112, 1175 (1966).

11 Fogelman, M.; Abbasi A. S.; Pearce, M. L.; Kattus, A. A.: Echocardiographic study of the abnormal motion of the posterior left ventricular wall during angina pectoris. Circulation *46:* 905–913 (1972).

12 Gregg, D. E.: in Luisada, Cardiovascular functions (McGraw Hill, New York 1962).

13 Hughes, M. L.; Mortensen, F.; Shourie, L.: Comparison of continuous and long-term heparin and anticoagulant therapy in patients with severe angina pectoris. Am. Heart J. *65:* 615–627 (1963).

14 Kattus, A.: Medical versus surgical therapy for ischemic heart disease. Chest *58:* suppl. I, pp. 299–304 (1970).

15 Kavanagh, T.; Shephard, R. J.; Chisholm, A. W.; Qureshi, S.; Kennedy, J.: Prognostic indexes for patients with ischemic heart disease enrolled in an exercise-centred rehabilitation program. Am. J. Cardiol. *44:* 1230–1240 (1979).

16 Kavanagh, T.; Shephard, R. J.: Conditioning of post-coronary patients. Comparison of continuous and interval training. Archs phys. Med. Rehabil. *56:* 72–76 (1975).

17 Kellermann, J. J.: Rehabilitation of patients with coronary heart disease. Prog. cardiovasc. Dis. *17:* 303–328 (1975).

18 Kellermann, J. J.; Ben-Ari, E.; Chayet, M.; Lapidot, C.; Drory, Y.; Fisman, E.: Cardiocirculatory response to different types of training in patients with angina pectoris. Cardiology *62:* 218–231 (1977).

19 Kennedy, C. K.; Spiekerman, R. E.; Lindsay, M. I.; Mankin, H. T.; Frye, R. L.; McCallister, B. D.: One year graduated exercise program for men with angina pectoris. Evaluation by physiological studies and coronary arteriography. Mayo Clin. Proc. *51:* 231–236 (1976).

20 Kitamura, K.; Jorgensen, C. R.; Gobel, F. L.; Taylor, H. L,; Wang, Y.: Haemodynamic correlates of myocardial oxygen consumption during upright exercise. J. appl. Physiol. *32:* 516–522 (1972).

21 McGregor, M.: Coronary steal, a review; in Roskamm, Reindell, Das chronisch kranke Herz, p. 69 (Schattauer, Stuttgart 1973).

22 Mirsky, I.; Ghista, D. N.; Sandler, H.: Cardiac mechanics; physiological clinical and mathematical considerations (Wiley/Interscience, New York 1974).

23 Moir, T. W.; Debra, D. W.: Effect of left ventricular hypertension, ischemia, and vasoactive drugs on the myocardial distribution of coronary flow. Circulation Res. *21:* 65–74 (1967).

24 Murphy, M. L.; Hultgren, H. N.; Detré, K.; Thomsen, J.; Takaro, T.: Treatment of chronic stable angina: a preliminary report of survival data of the randomized Veterans Administration Cooperative Study; in Pollock, Schmidt, Heart disease and rehabilitation, pp. 228–242 (Houghton Mifflin, Boston 1979).

25 Parker, J. O.; di Giorgi, S.; West, R. O.: A haemodynamic study of acute coronary insufficiency precipitated by exercise. With observations on the effects of nitroglycerin. Am. J. Med. *17:* 470–483 (1966).

26 Redwood, D. R.; Rosing, D. R.; Epstein S. E.: Circulatory and symptomatic effects of physical training in patients with coronary artery disease and angina pectoris. New Engl. J. Med. *286:* 959–965 (1972).

27 Robin, E.; Cowan, C.; Puri, P.; Ganguly, S.; DeBoyrie, E.; Martinez, M.; Stock, T.; Bing, R. J.: A comparative study of nitroglycerin and propranolol. Circulation *36:* 175–186 (1967).

28 Shephard, R. J.: Recurrence of myocardial infarction in an exercising population. Br. Heart J. *42:* 133–138 (1979).

29 Sim, D. N.; Neill, W. A.: Investigation of the physiological basis for increased exercise threshold for angina pectoris after physical conditioning. J. clin. Invest. *54:* 763–770 (1974).

30 Smith, J. L.; Dressendorfer, R. H.; Amsterdam, E. A.: Evaluation of a walking program for patients with ischemic heart disease (IHD). Beneficial effects without increased maximal oxygen uptake ($\dot{V}_{O_2max}$). Med. Sci. Sports *11:* 100 (1979).

31 Stevenson, J. A. F.: Exercise, food intake and health in experimental animals. Can. med. Ass. J. *96:* 862–866 (1967).

32 Tauchert, M.; Kochsiek, K.; Heiss, H. W.; Strauer, B. E.; Kettler, D.; Reploh, H. D.; Rau, G.; Bretschneider, H. J.: Measurement of coronary blood flow in man by the argon method; in Maseri, Myocardial blood flow in man. Methods and significance in coronary disease, pp. 139–144 (Minerva Medica, Torino 1972).

33 Trap-Jensen, J.; Clausen, J. P.: Effect of training on the relation of heart rate and blood pressure to the onset of pain in effort angina pectoris; in Larsen, Malmborg, Coronary heart disease and physical fitness (Munksgaard, Copenhagen 1971).

34 Varnauskas, E.; Holmberg, S.: Myocardial blood flow during exercise in patients with coronary heart disease. Comments on training effects; in Larsen, Malmborg, Coronary heart disease and physical fitness, pp. 102–104 (University Park Press, Baltimore 1971).

35 Wenger, N. K.: Does exercise training enhance collateral circulation? in Kellermann, Denolin, Critical evaluation of cardiac rehabilitation, pp. 143–145 (Karger, Basel 1977).

36 Zohman, L. R.; Tobis, J. S.: The effect of exercise training on patients with angina pectoris. Phys. Med. *48:* 525–532 (1967).

Dr. R. J. Shephard, 320 Huron Street, Toronto, Ont. M5S 1A1 (Canada)

Adv. Cardiol., vol. 31, pp. 199–204 (Karger, Basel 1982)

Is Strenuous Physical Activity Appropriate for Patients with Coronary Heart Disease?[1]

Nanette K. Wenger

Emory University School of Medicine, Atlanta, Ga., USA

The concept of individualized prescriptive physical activity is central to rehabilitative exercise training for patients with coronary atherosclerotic heart disease [1]. Because of the heterogeneity of patients with symptomatic coronary disease and their major qualitative and quantitative differences in functional impairment, recommendations for physical activity must be based on the results of exercise testing. Indeed, the exercise test is ideally performed with the patient receiving the drug regimen to be maintained during training. Patients with coronary disease should never perform at an activity level greater than that safely completed, i.e., without adverse signs or symptoms, at a recent exercise test. Exercise testing [7] permits quantitative determination of the patient's functional capacity and hemodynamic response to exercise; it defines the level of activity at which evidence of myocardial ischemia and/or arrhythmias may occur [3].

Strenuous Physical Activity

The dictionary definition of strenuous is 'vigorous activity; energetic, calling for physical energy or stamina; arduous; rigorous'. However, in determining whether strenuous activity is appropriate or inappropriate for the coronary patient, we must appreciate that 'strenuous' exertion is not an absolute, but rather relates to the patient's preinfarction activity level, to

[1] Adapted from Wenger, N.K.: Patients with coronary heart disease should avoid strenuous physical exertion: Antagonist position; in Rapaport, Current controversies in cardiovascular disease (Saunders, Philadelphia 1980), with permission.

the preinfarction physical fitness of the patient, and to the extent of residual physiologic impairment after myocardial infarction.

Realistic Goals of Exercise Training

A review of the realistic goals of exercise training enables the assessment of whether strenuous physical activity is appropriate or warranted. Although exercise training has a number of beneficial effects, there is no definitive evidence that it alters the natural history of coronary disease – reinfarction, sudden death, or total mortality – or that it increases the coronary collateral circulation.

A realistic goal for patients after myocardial infarction in an exercise training program is improvement of physical work capacity and work efficiency [3, 8]. The physiologic response to training [1, 5, 6], in patients after myocardial infarction as well as in normal individuals, is characterized by a modest decrease in the resting heart rate and systolic blood pressure and by a faster return to normal of the heart rate after exercise. More important, there is a lesser increase in heart rate and systolic blood pressure for any level of submaximal work. These latter two parameters, the rate-pressure product, or 'double product', are major determinants of myocardial oxygen demand. It is thus expected that the trained coronary patient, with a lesser myocardial oxygen demand for any submaximal task, will have less or no angina pectoris, and less or no ST-segment displacement on the electrocardiogram, as evidence of myocardial ischemia, than was the case prior to training. This is the mechanism for improvement in work efficiency. An additional physiologic benefit of exercise training is an increase in maximal oxygen uptake; this is due to augmentation of the blood supply to exercising muscle and to improved oxygen extraction. There is increasing evidence that high-level, long-term training may also improve myocardial function and/or oxygen supply, but this is not observed with the usual moderate exercise currently recommended and feasible for most patients recovered from myocardial infarction. These are the mechanisms by which training improves exercise tolerance and decreases symptoms of myocardial ischemia, permitting a greater intensity and duration of both occupational and recreational activity before attainment of the patient's ischemic threshold [6, 8]. With exercise training, many patients after myocardial infarction can not only be restored to their preinfarction status, but can achieve a level of fitness greater than that prior to their illness.

Exercise may also exert a favorable effect on other and possibly more powerful coronary risk factors. It aids in weight control, may provide an incentive for the cessation of cigarette smoking, and is associated with a decrease in serum triglyceride level. Although the effect on total serum cholesterol level is variable, the HDL cholesterol appears increased. Insufficient data are available to evaluate the effect of physical activity on platelet aggregation or fibrinolysis; similarly, data remain controversial regarding the effect of exercise on cardiac arrhythmias. Improvement in psychologic status is of particular importance, in that there is more impairment after infarction from emotional than physiologic problems. Patients who exercise and become physically fit feel better, have an improved self-image, have lessened anxiety and depression scores as measured on standard psychometric tests, and appear better able to tolerate life stresses. Exercise appears to aid patients in renouncing the sick role and returning to a normal life-style, including return to work.

Prescriptive Components of Exercise [2, 3]

Exercise training requires the imposition of a target workload which is a calculated percentage of the patient's measured physical work capacity. To achieve a training effect, patients should exercise at least 2 or 3 times weekly, preferrably on nonsuccessive days; and for a 30- to 45-min session that includes a warm-up and cool-down period. The intensity recommended is 70–85% of the highest heart rate safely achieved at prior exercise testing [7]. Although somewhat arbitrary, these recommendations are generally considered effective, in that they correspond to 60–78% of the peak oxygen uptake, an adequate yet safe challenge to the oxygen transport system.

Exercise [2] should be dynamic, involving the rhythmic, repetitive movements of large muscle groups; and both arms and legs should be trained, as their training effects are only minimally interchangeable. Isotonic exercise increases the heart rate, stroke volume and cardiac output proportionate to the intensity of the activity, with little associated change in mean arterial blood pressure. The sustained increase in blood flow required to meet the metabolic needs of large masses of exercising muscle places an increased volume load on the heart, inducing the conditioning or training effect. Interval training is recommended to avoid incurring an oxygen debt. Isotonic activities include walking, jogging, swimming, bicycling, noncompetitive running games, and cross-country skiing.

Myocardial Infarction: Residual Physiologic Impairment [6, 8]

Let us relate these desirable features of prescriptive exercise to the residual physiologic impairment which may be encountered in the patient who has sustained a myocardial infarction. The degree of physiologic impairment relates to the amount of myocardial necrosis and scarring, to the site of infarction, and to the presence and amount of residual ischemic myocardium. Whereas congestive heart failure is virtually absent in patients with angina pectoris in the absence of myocardial infarction, most patients with greater than a 20% infarction of the left ventricle have evidence of congestive heart failure. The clinically familiar New York Heart Association functional classification enables some general guidelines regarding physical activity to be developed.

About 50% of patients remain in functional class I after an initial myocardial infarction. These patients are asymptomatic at ordinary levels of daily vocational and leisure activity; they have minimal or no functional cardiac impairment, and typically have neither angina pectoris, congestive heart failure, nor serious arrhythmia. Because less than 5% of myocardium is infarcted, they can readily perform at workloads of 7–8 mets or greater, and thus have virtually no occupational or physical activity restrictions. These patients, with little or no detectable alteration of cardiac performance can and do participate in high-level recreational physical activities; marathon running and other 'strenuous' activities are quite appropriate for a subset of these individuals when properly trained [9].

Class II patients become symptomatic with prolonged physical and/or emotional stress because they have a 20–40% impairment of cardiac function. However, they have an occupational or recreational tolerance in the 4–5 MET range and thus can be expected to perform most general industrial labor.

Class III individuals become symptomatic with usual daily living activities because of their 50–75% impairment of cardiac function. Their exercise tolerance is usually limited to the 3–4 MET range. They are not candidates for 'strenuous' physical activity, unless their functional capacity can be improved by medical and/or surgical intervention. Vocationally, most desk or bench jobs are within their capabilities. Nevertheless, low-level prescriptive exercise training may be appropriate for selected patients, with careful monitoring of their myocardial ischemic threshold, of the appearance of or increase in arrhythmias, and the exacerbation of left ventricular dysfunction or congestive heart failure.

The severely impaired class IV patients are symptomatic at rest or with minimal activity; their impairment of cardiac function is greater than 80%, explaining their functional capacity of 2 METS or less. Symptoms may be those of myocardial ischemia (angina pectoris), congestive heart failure, arrhythmia, or a combination of these problems. Their vocational capabilities are extremely limited, and even moderate levels of physical activity are inappropriate.

Obviously, then, activity prescription is related significantly both to the degree of cardiac functional impairment and to preinfarction activity levels. For example, for the executive who (prior to myocardial infarction) never performed activity more demanding than swiveling in a desk chair, the prescription of bicycling, tennis, or golf, exercise in the 3–5 MET range, would represent a modest increase in cardiac work; and snow-shoveling or skiing (6–7 METS) would constitute a considerable activity increment. But the laborer whose typical activity is digging ditches, carrying heavy loads, etc., i.e., one whose occupational work level is 7–8 METS or greater, can readily be expected to jog, play basketball, canoe, etc. if there is not significant residual physiologic impairment from the infarction. This emphasizes the importance of the prior level or performance and fitness.

Benefits of Physical Activity

The basic principle underlying prescription of physical activity for the coronary patient involves determination of a safe and effective workload. This is one which can achieve a training effect with a minimal risk of myocardial ischemia and/or orthopedic complications [3, 4]. The proper approach, then, is not to question whether 'strenuous' physical exertion is appropriate or inappropriate for the patient with symptomatic coronary disease, but rather to identify the beneficial and safe absolute workload for an individual coronary patient at a specific stage in recovery and rehabilitation. This concept maximizes the benefits of exercise training without imposition of undue hazard.

Substantial benefits can accrue when individualized prescriptive physical activity is incorporated into the plan of care for selected patients after myocardial infarction. Favorable responses include an improved functional capacity and work performance, decreased symptoms of myocardial ischemia, reduced psychologic impairment, and an enhanced return to vocational and leisure activities [1, 6, 8].

References

1 Mitchell, J. H.: Exercise training in the treatment of coronary heart disease. Adv. intern. Med. *20:* 249 (1975).

2 Haskell, W. L.: Design and implementation of cardiac conditioning programs: in Wenger, Hellerstein, Rehabilitation of the coronary patient, p. 203 (Wiley, New York 1978).

3 The Exercise Standard Book: American Heart Association, 70-041-A, Dallas, Texas, 1979.

4 Haskell, W. L.: Cardiovascular complications during exercise training of cardiac patients. Circulation *57:* 920 (1978).

5 Saltin, B.: The interplay between peripheral and central factors in the adaptive response to exercise and training. Ann. N. Y. Acad. Sci. *301:* 224 (1977).

6 Paterson, D. H.; Shephard, R. J.; Cunningham, D.; Jones, N. L.; Andrew, G.: Effects of physical training on cardiovascular function following myocardial infarction. J. appl. Physiol. *47:* 482 (1979).

7 Naughton, J.; Haider, R.: Methods of exercise testing; in Naughton, Hellerstein, Mohler, Exercise testing and exercise training in coronary heart disease, p. 79 (Academic Press, New York 1973).

8 Verani, M. S.; Hartung, G, H.; Hoepfel-Harris, J.; Welton, D. E.; Pratt, C. M.; Miller, R. R.: Effects of exercise training on left ventricular performance and myocardial perfusion in patients with coronary artery disease. Am. J. Cardiol. *47:* 797 (1981).

9 Hellerstein, H. K.: Limitations of marathon running in the rehabilitation of coronary patients: anatomic and physiologic determinants. Ann. N. Y. Acad. Sci. *301:* 484 (1978).

N. K. Wenger, MD, Emory University School of Medicine,
Thomas K. Glenn Memorial Building, 69 Butler Street, S. E., Atlanta, GA 30303 (USA)

Adv. Cardiol., vol. 31, pp. 205–211 (Karger, Basel 1982)

Practical Aspects of Vigorous Exercise Programming for Coronary Patients

L. R. Zohman

Montefiore Hospital and Medical Center, Bronx, N. Y., USA

Numerous articles have appeared in the literature during the past 10 years presenting guidelines for prescription of aerobic activities, for both normal and cardiac subjects. Self-monitoring of heart rate by patients is familiar and physicians can now recognize the trained state. However, sophistication in exercise programming brings with it additional, more complex, less easily answered questions. This presentation hopes to offer a viewpoint on: (1) exercise programming for the more impaired or more risky patient; (2) day-to-day management of the exercising cardiac, and (3) how to develop a cardiac exercise group.

Exercise Programming for the More-Impaired Patient

Although left ventricular dysfunction, ventricular dysrhythmias or recent myocardial infarction are usually considered contraindications to exercise training, exercise is being prescribed at times in all these conditions.

Patients with *ejection fractions below 40%* can be trained and may achieve both peripheral muscular and psychological benefit without improved myocardial function, or further deterioration [1]. In the study of *Froelicher* et al. [2], 5 of 16 coronary heart disease patients with left ventricular dysfunction on exercise, who were evaluated using nuclide studies before and after 3–12 months of exercise training, actually showed improvement in both ejection fraction and thallium images and reached higher treadmill workloads at the same rate-pressure products. Therefore, it is no longer mandatory to exclude patients with impaired left ventricular function from exercise. Training may or may not improve myocardial contractility, but it probably will do no harm.

Individuals with *complex ventricular arrhythmias* (such as couplets or short runs of ventricular tachycardia) occurring on high level exercise but without cardiac disease are no longer either being excluded from exercise training or being treated with maintenance antiarrhythmics unless one can document that there is a re-entry pathway [3].

However, complex arrhythmias occurring at <70% maximal heart rate or <130 BPM among 'normal' individuals suggest that evaluation is needed to confirm the absence of coronary disease [4]. When patients with ventricular arrhythmias also have ischemic exercise tests and presumably left ventricular dysfunction, anti-arrhythmic therapy is indicated although it may fail to alter the situation in 65% of the cases [5]. If therapy leaves the patient with simple ventricular ectopy, exercise training may decrease the frequency of these VPBs [6].

In management, it is useful to determine whether the arrhythmias appeared only during vigorous effort since they may be prevented by avoiding that much effort. Or, exercise recommendations might stress unusually long, gradual warm-up and cool-down periods. Among coronary patients, even those without ischemia on exercise electrocardiography, sometimes a nitroglycerin tablet immediately before exercise may prevent the problem.

The *high risk patient* for exercise programming is one who is markedly ischemic at low work levels on the treadmill test. However, once placed on maximal medical therapy (if inoperable) he may profit from conditioning under supervision, or he may carry out a walking program if unsupervised. He should exercise at the time of peak action of his medication, at least 2 h after a meal, when he is least tired, and often pretreated by nitroglycerin. Providing the patient with information about the effects of environmental temperature and sudden effort, and symptoms requiring medical evaluation is important.

Early exercise training, 3 weeks after infarction has been used without ill effects [7] based on the assumption that small infarcts heal within 3 weeks, and the observations that nuclide studies show no worse left ventricular function among early exercisers than controls, and rehabilitation is shortened. It remains to be discerned whether such early training augments collateralization or decreases the number of arrhythmic deaths which occur between weeks 3 and 11.

Day-to-Day Management of the Exercising Cardiac

The *pulse counting* ritual identifies the cardiac exercise class; yet there is little uniformity in how this procedure is carried out or used. After one report [8] carotid counts became suspect since carotid sinus pressure might not only be dangerous, but might falsely lower the counts obtained. Subsequent studies have shown that carotid counts are simple, safe and reliable in most cases [9].

The question of whether to start counting from 'zero' or 'one' is a matter of intradisciplinary preference, the exercise physiologists starting with 'zero' and the cardiologists with 'one'. My own view favors starting the count with 'one' for practical reasons. Since it takes the patient several seconds to find his pulse and start counting as the rate slows down, this falsely low count balances the slightly higher value obtained by starting the count with 'one'. In our program, heart rate counts started with 'one' check closely with telemetered ECG rates.

For practical reasons too (simplicity) we use the American Heart Association (AHA) method rather than the Karvonen method of determining target heart rate. The Karvonen formula provides a heart rate range by subtracting the resting heart rate from the maximal rate and patients exercise at 40–60% of this range above the resting heart rate. The AHA recommendations are 70–85% of the maximal attainable heart rate rather than heart rate range, e. g., a 50-year-old man might have a maximal heart rate of 170 with a target zone of 119–145 bpm according to AHA guidelines. Depending on his resting heart rate he might have a Karvonen target pulse rate of from 90 to 130 bpm. Since the resting heart rate is influenced by so many noncardiac factors, and there is no definitive evidence for the superiority of the Karvonen method, our preference is to use the AHA guidelines and begin exercise programming at the 70% of maximum heart rate level.

Pulse rates both at rest and during exercise are lowered by *beta blockade* so that the target heart rate prescription must be modified accordingly. One way is to determine the maximal heart rate from the exercise test carried out on propranolol calculating the 70–85% zone from this measured maximum. Alternatively, if oxygen consumption is measured, during the stress test, the heart rate at 60–80% of the maximal oxygen consumption achieved can be assigned as a target [10] since oxygen consumption will not be changed by administration of propranolol. Or, some exercise training programs arbitrarily set the upper training heart rate at 10 beats less than the maximal rate achieved on the exercise test on beta blockade.

A more important question is whether patients do, in fact, achieve a training effect if they train on a beta blocker. To date, this question has not been resolved. *Hellerstein* et al. [11] tested 1 patient on and off propranolol on a monthly basis and trained him on beta blocker. On propranolol, exercise could proceed to higher workloads after training but this improvement disappeared when the patient exercised off medication. *Obma* et al. [12] tested cardiac subjects both on and off propranolol and trained them on propranolol and *Lester and Wallace* [13] used the same protocol for pairs of normal subjects (one per pair as a non-blocker control). Results showed no impairment of the ability to train on beta blockade. However, both studies suffer from a lack of proof that the patients were maximally beta-blocked. Similarly, our own findings show that training can be achieved when cardiac patients are not maximally blocked [14]. Whether training can result when patients are maximally blocked is unknown but seems unlikely.

Day-to-day management requires recommending a *program entry level* in terms of activity as well as heart rate target zone. Some suggestions follow:

Walking: (a) Start at speed on level ground that subject reached at 10% grade on the treadmill test, or (b) start at 2.0 mph if completed Bruce Stage I, 3.0 mph if completed II, 4.0 mph if completed III.

Stationary cycling: Start 150 kp below maximal level reached on bicycle test, interval pattern.

Stairs: Up 2 flights, walk 100 feet or walk down 2 flights, repeat 3 times.

Calisthenics: Use entry level about ⅔ of MET capacity achieved on stress test or lower level as warm-up (seated exercises approximately 2 METS, standing including arms approximately 2–3, leg lifting approximately 3–4 [15].

Aerobic dancing: Use entry level about ⅔ of MET level achieved on exercise test (low level = approx. 4 METS; mid level = approx. 6 METS; high level = approx. 8 METS) [16].

Progressing on an exercise program may be considered when there is symptomatic improvement without signs of musculoskeletal overuse and the heart rate response to the present exercise challange is below the target heart rate zone. The duration of the activity should first be lengthened (double the walking distance at the same workload; add two flights of stairs/week at same climbing rate; increase the number or repetitions of the same calisthenics or dance for twice the time). Then the intensity should be increased (walk faster; increase bicycle resistance; dance at mid versus low level, etc.) for a somewhat shorter duration. Then again increase duration. Progressing to the next step depends on being below target heart rate on repeated measurements.

Kavanagh [17] has developed a progressing heart rate nomogram which permits one to assess when exercise may be increased by connecting a resting heart rate scale with the maximal heart rate scale. The progressing heart rate read from a third scale is approximately 70% of maximal heart rate.

Boredom is often a management problem. A patient may switch to other types of exercise programs entirely or may use circuit training in which he sequentially does various activities – stationary cycling, lifting of light weights (many repetitions), jumping rope, jogging in place, calisthenics, stair climbing, all of which may be done in his own home. A home bicycle may be used both for pedalling and for arm cranking.

Program Development for Groups of Cardiac Patients

Cardiac exercise groups provide camaraderie, supervision, economy of physician time and the possibility of adding other risk factor control services.

The best plan is to *keep start-up costs down* by (1) using existing testing equipment; (2) buying exercise training equipment last since fitness activities can be used which require no equipment, e. g., jogging; (3) use part-time staffing on a per session basis, or employees who can serve dual functions; (4) provide reimbursible services first to generate income, adding nonreimbursible services when profits can support them, and (5) minimize physician time since his services are costly.

The latter can be done by carrying out testing and training simultaneously (if medical supervision is needed) or when the physician is on the premises. Or, trained physical educators can supervise maintenance cardiac exercise classes. Having physicians or nurses in exercise classes is neither cost effective nor necessary [18]. Average mortality in cardiac exercise classes as reported in a survey by *Haskell* [19] is one death per 212,182 patient hours in recent years.

In organizing a program, the responsible individual should familiarize himself with all available literature on exercise testing, prescription and training. Mail surveys and visits to other programs are usually not useful since the information is generally not transferable to developing the new program. It is preferable to decide on the needs of a particular community, staff availability, sources of patient referrals and to build the program to fit the situation. Telephone or mail inquiries to experts about specific program problems are willingly handled if they do not impose needlessly for background information which should have been sought out on one's own. Programs should be developed by one interested physician as leader-supervisor with the support of a medical advisory panel to assure the broadest possible community acceptance and referral base.

Lastly, it does not seem wise to buy *commercially developed testing and training programs* although they can provide early guidance, since ultimately their 'royalties' may prove excessive. Their pattern of operation may not be appropriate for a particular community. Large cash outlays for equipment are also inadvisable so that lease-purchase agreements and modular equipment which can be expanded can suffice. In fact, an ECG machine, defibrillator and 'know how' are all that is needed to start a program.

References

1 Lee, A. P.; Ice, R.; Blessey, R.; Sanmarco, M. E.: Long-term effects of physical training on coronary patients with impaired ventricular function. Circulation *60:* 1519 (1979).

2 Froelicher, V.; Jensen, D.; Atwood, J. E.; McKirnan, M. D.; Gerber, K.; Slutsky, R.; Battler, A.; Ashburn, W.; Ross, J., Jr.: Cardiac rehabilitation. Evidence for improvement in myocardial perfusion and function. Archs phys. Med. Rehabil. *65:* 517 (1980).

3 Margolis, B.; DeSilva, R. A.; Lown, B.: Episodic drug treatment in the management of paroxysmal arrhythmias. Am. J. Cardiol. *45:* 621 (1980).

4 McHenry, P. L.; Morris, S. N.; Kavalier, M.; Jordan, J. W.: Comparative study of exercise-induced ventricular arrhythmias in normal subjects and patients with documented coronary artery disease. Am. J. Cardiol. *37:* 609 (1976).

5 Goldschlager, N.; Cohn, K.; Goldschlager, A.: Exercise-related ventricular arrhythmias. Mod. Concepts cardiovasc. Dis. *XLVIII:* 67 (1979).

6 Blackburn, H.; Taylor, H. L.; Hamrell, B.; Buskirk, E.; Nicholas, W. C.; Thorsen, R. D.: Premature ventricular complexes induced by stress testing. Their frequency and response to physical conditioning. Am. J. Cardiol. *31:* 441 (1973).

7 DeBusk, R. E.; Houston, N.; Haskell, W.; Fry, G.; Parker, M.: Exercise training soon after myocardial infarction. Am. J. Cardiol. *44:* 1223 (1979).

8 White, J. R.: EKG changes using carotid artery for heart rate monitoring. Med. Sci. Sports *9:* 88 (1977).

9 Oldridge, N. B.; Haskell, W. L.; Single, P.: Carotid palpation, coronary heart disease and exercise rehabilitation. Med. Sci. Sports Exer. *13:* 6 (1981).

10 Zohman, L. R.: Beyond diet: exercise your way to fitness and heart health, CPC International, Englewood Cliffs 1974, p. 14. (Single copies available gratis from Department ZJH, Box 307, Coventry, CT 06238, USA).
11 Hellerstein, H. K.; Hirsch, E. Z.; Ader, R.; Greenblott, N.; Siegel, M.: Principles of exercise prescription for normal and cardiac subjects; in Naughton, Hellerstein, Mohler, Exercise testing and exercise training in coronary heart disease, p. 163 (Academic Press, New York 1973).
12 Obma, R. T.; Wilson, P. K.; Goebel, M. E.; Campbell, D. E.: Effect of a conditioning program in patients taking propranolol for angina pectoris. Cardiology *64:* 365 (1979).
13 Lester, R. M.; Wallace, A. G.: Cardiovascular adaptations to beta adrenergic blockade during physical training (Abstract No. 545). Circulation *57:* II–140 (1978).
14 Zohman, L. R.; Kattus, A. A.: Cardiac rehabilitation for the practicing physician, p. 56 (Stratton Intercontinental Medical Book Corp., New York 1979).
15 Greer, M.; Weber, T.; Dimick, S.; Ratliff, R.: Physiological responses to low-intensity cardiac rehabilitation exercises. Phys. Ther. *60:* 1146 (1980).
16 Zohman, L. R.; Kattus, A. A.; Softness, D.: The cardiologists' guide to fitness and health through exercise, p. 167 (Simon & Schuster, New York 1979).
17 Kavanagh, T.: Heart attack, counterattack, p. 122 (Van Nostrand Reinhold, Toronto 1976).
18 Zohman, L. R.; Kattus, A. A.: Cardiac rehabilitation for the practicing physician, p. 59 (Stratton Intercontinental Medical Book Corp., New York 1979).
19 Haskell, W. L.: Cardiovascular complications during medically supervised exercise training; in Cohen, Mock, Ringqvist, Physical conditioning and cardiovascular rehabilitation, p. 159 (Wiley, New York 1981).

L. R. Zohman, MD, Montefiore Hospital and Medical Center,
111 East 210 Street, Bronx, NY 10467 (USA)

Adv. Cardiol., vol. 31, pp. 212–217 (Karger, Basel 1982)

Coping with Cardiac Disease[1]

Thomas P. Hackett, Ned H. Cassem

Psychiatric Consultation-Liaison Service, Department of Psychiatry, Massachusetts General Hospital, Boston, Mass., USA

The concept of coping is one that has received much attention in the psychological literature of late, and, to a lesser extent, in medical journals as well [1]. 'To cope' is taken from the French verb 'couper', which means to slash or strike. Essentially, it means the ability to fight back. Although the notion is simple enough, there is some confusion at the present time because coping has become entwined with the Freudian concept of the defense mechanism.

Coping, in contrast to the defense mechanism, has from its beginning been associated with normal rather than neurotic mechanisms. While all of us use defense mechanisms, these are rarely discussed. In contrast, frequent reference is made to man's ability to cope. To be able to call upon normal and effective coping tactics or mechanisms is a sign of maturity and good mental health. Perhaps the most important thing about coping that has come to light is that many of these tactics can be taught. If not taught, certain tendencies that have to do with adequate or good coping can be encouraged.

A number of studies have demonstrated that the first response of most North Americans to chest pain is to act in such a way that the average delay is between 4 and 5 hours [2, 3]. This pattern of behavior seems to bear no relationship to educational level, socioeconomic class, sex, the history of

[1] Work prepared under Contract PHS 43-67-1443 and HE 13781 of National Institutes of Health, Public Health Service, United States Department of Health, Education and Welfare.

previous myocardial infarction (MI), acquaintance with individuals who have had angina and cardiovascular disease, or those who have been exposed to an educational program in which these principles are outlined. This delay is an example of maladaptive coping. Perhaps in response to the implicit threat that chest pain is related to the possibility of sudden death, the victim tends to rationalize or explain his pain on the basis of some less lethal symptom. He most often displaces the pain from the heart to the stomach. This type of response bears little or no relationship to logic and seems to resist all attempts at education.

What is the root of this delay? It is caused in part by a mechanism called denial. Denial is a defense mechanism. We chose to use these terms – coping tactic and defense mechanism – interchangeably. The defense of denial was originally described by *Anna Freud* [4]. She dealt largely with children and described their denial by word, act, and fantasy. Denial is now used by psychiatrists to describe a way of blindly avoiding confrontations with dangerous fantasies, thoughts, situations, or persons. It can take place on an unconscious or conscious level [5]. We define denial as the repudiation of part or all of the total available meaning of an event in order to minimize or reduce anxiety [6]. There are, however, two aspects of denial. One is the process of denying, and the other is the result of that process, or the fact of denial. Most defense mechanisms, whether they are intellectualization, rationalization, repudiation, or others, have as their goal the minimization of fear. Thus, all defense mechanisms can be seen as means to effect a denial of fear or its counterpart. Along with these many mechanisms is the defense of denial itself, which is simply the failure to perceive, interpret or understand the full meaning of an event. For example, perceptual denial of chest pain might result in a so-called silent coronary.

Weisman [6] defines denial as consisting of four successive steps. First, the symptom itself or the threatening problem has to be accepted. The second step is based upon repudiation of a portion of the accepted meaning. The third is replacement of the repudiated portion with a more congenial version. The fourth is reorientation of the individual to accommodate the revised reality. Thus, the individual with chest pain would have to accept the chest pain as a fact. Step No. 2 would involve the repudiation of a portion of the meaning of the pain. He would thus displace the source from heart to stomach. In step No. 3, he would replace the meaning with a more congenial version; thus, he would say, from in the stomach it must be indigestion. No. 4, he would reorient his behavior to accommodate the revised reality by taking an antacid.

Denial also implies the lack of introspective brooding about the future. The patient must be able to either forget about worries or to reduce their magnitude. This is particularly important for physicians to understand, because doctors are the best agents for providing hope and optimism. The real problems, as we see them, are in cardiac convalescence and in the rehabilitation of the post-MI patient. This is where the doctors's attitude becomes so important.

Psychological problems found in individuals who are recovering from an MI are generally centered around two states of mind, depression and anxiety. These conditions generally come in the same package. They are part and parcel of the same response. Anxiety generally stems from the threath of sudden death, and depression centers around the question of whether the patient can function successfully as a spouse, parent, and citizen. Also, the MI patient generally feels as though he has lost a part of himself. Usually it is a valued part, such as strength, energy and independence. A subjective sense of depletion, along with weakness and easy fatigue, are characteristic of the individuals in the first post-MI month.

When the patient is about to be discharged from the hospital following an uncomplicated MI, he generally has a fairly good state of mind. His worries are confined to realistic aspects, and he is glad to be returning home. Once he has arrived home, as a result of bed rest and inactivity, the patient experiences a sense of weakness which dogs his every activity. It is as though his body is not up to the tasks that the thought it was. He nearly always interprets this incorrectly as a sign that this heart is worse off than he was told. The symptom of easy fatigue and weakness herald the onset of what we have termed the 'homecoming depression' [7]. Most patients are able to weather the discouragement of the early weeks at home without disrupting their lives or the lives of their families. However, we all know that the post-MI patient during early convalescence at home is besieged with many psychological difficulties. The patient is apt to feel unprotected and vulnerable after the close scrutiny he was given in the hospital. Furthermore, the severe restrictions placed on smoking, eating, and the use of alcohol are discouraging, and these are compounded by questions about activities – sexual, social, and physical – which cause worry. In addition, there are also a variety of common misconceptions surrounding coronary artery disease. These are deep-rooted myths that tend to resist all attempts to extricate them. Since these misconceptions are best dispelled by education from the physician, we will list them:

(a) Even mild exercise is dangerous.

(b) Sexual intercourse should never be attempted, because following an MI one is 'over the hill'.

(c) Repeated infarctions or sudden death is more likely to occur at sexual orgasm.

(d) Driving must be avoided.

(e) The arms must not be suddenly raised over the head, especially the left arm.

(f) The patient is apt to die at the same age as the parent who had heart disease.

(g) Recurrence is apt to take place around the anniversary of the first infarction.

(h) The heart is more vulnerable to repeat infarctions and sudden death while the patient sleeps.

If one looks to the model of providing maximum coping ability for the problems of cardiac convalescence, the physician could fashion a program around five crucial points. The first of these would be clearing up misconceptions through *education.* Since patients will rarely volunteer these beliefs, it is best for the physician to bring them up himself, specifically asking the patient if he has ever had such ideas as those listed from (a) through (h). Although these beliefs are more common in blue-collar populations, they occur across all strata of society. Queries about sex are more commonly made by the educated. Patients from lower socioeconomic backgrounds are often too embarrassed to speak of sex.

The best time to detoxify and clarify misconceptions and to impart the facts is just before the patient leaves the hospital. It is important to set aside half an hour or more to chat with the patient and his wife. Point by point the doctor should discuss medications, activities, diet, various restrictions, and also the tendency of the family to overprotect and baby the patient. With the couple alone, advice should be given about sexual performance. Good articles are available on this topic. Liberal use should also be made of the excellent pamphlets and booklets offered by the American Heart Association.

The second point is *anticipation.* The post-MI depression, called the 'homecoming depression', can be reduced in intensity if the patient is warned about the sense of tiredness and easy fatigue he may experience upon returning home. He should be told this does not mean his heart is failing but that it is a natural response to the inactivity of bedrest. He should also be warned to expect anxiety when he increases his range of activities, and particularly around the time that he returns to work. If anxiety and depression are anticipated and identified as normal responses, the patient is inclined to feel less alone with these unpleasant emotions, less unusual.

The third crucial point is *medication*. Recurrent anxiety is best handled by determining its cause and by offering explanations and reassurances when these are in order. However, tranquilizers should be used in conjunction with counselling. They are often valuable in maintaining equanimity. Tranquilizers for the chronically anxious should be awarded the same importance as cardiac drugs. The benzodiazepines are a safe group of tranquilizers for cardiac patients. Generally the dosage schedule is as follows: diazepam (Valium) 2–5 mg, chlordiazepoxide (Librium) 5–10 mg, or oxazepam (Serax) 15 mg, 3 or 4 times a day. Because many patients will regard regular pill-taking as being unmanly, the doctor should stress the importance of following a regular regime and emphasize that the use of tranquilizers casts no aspersion on manhood. The use of tricyclic antidepressants requires special care in the early convalescent phase because of associated disturbances of heart rate and rhythm. These, along with the phenothiazines, have been implicated in sudden deaths. The use of monoamine oxidase inhibitors also requires care during convalescence from an MI because of the danger of hypertensive crises when tyramine-containing food is ingested. Sleep disturbances can be treated, particularly in the first month at home, with a hypnotic. The most convenient method of doing this is to double the dose of a benzodiazepine given for daytime sedation. Flurazepam (Dalmane) is a popular hypnotic, largely due to its reputed failure to suppress REM sleeping. The usual adult dosage is 30 mg at bedtime.

The fourth crucial point is *activity and physical conditioning*. There is little question that setting out a program of activity, which should be accompanied by a program of physical conditioning, is an excellent antidote for depression and seems to serve as a prophylaxis against this disorder of mood [8].

The fifth point concerns *relaxation techniques*. The use of relaxation states has strong attraction for certain individuals, but, like jogging, has a limited appeal for the majority. Nonetheless, the patient should be taught relaxation and/or autohypnosis in order to make these practices available should the patient choose to use them. Relaxation and activity both offer the patient a chance to take a hand in his own recovery. This, in turn, provides a sense of independence that is vital to some individuals.

The bottom line for coping is common sense. This, along with education and support, are the most important qualities that can be provided by the physician in his effort to help the patient through the experience of illness. The kind of advice the physician gives, along with his attitude and his ability to impart optimism and a sense of caring, can be lifesaving.

References

1 Coelho, G. V.; Hamburg, D. A.; Adams, J. E. (eds.): Coping and adaptation (Basic Books, New York 1974).

2 Hackett, T. P.; Cassem, N. H.: Factors contributing to delay in responding to the signs and symptoms of acute myocardial infarction. Am. J. Cardiol. *24:* 651 (1969).

3 Moss, A. J.; et al.: Delay in hospitalization during the acute coronary period. Am. J. Cardiol. *24:* 659 (1969).

4 Freud, A.: The ego and the mechanisms of defense. Translated by C. Baines (Hogarth Press Institute of Psychoanalysis, London 1948).

5 Weisman, A. D.: On dying and denying: a psychiatrist study of terminality (Behavioral Publications, New York 1972).

6 Weisman, A. D.; Hackett, T. P.: Predilection to death. Psychosom. Med. *23:* 232–255 (1961).

7 Wishnie, H. A.; Hackett, T. P.; Cassem, N. H.: Psychological hazards of convalescence following myocardial infarction. J. Am. med. Ass. *215:* 1292 (1971).

8 Hackett, T. P.; Cassem, N. H.: Psychological aspects of rehabilitation after myocardial infarction; in Wenger, Hellerstein, Rehabilitation of the patient after myocardial infarction, chapter 10 (Wiley & Sons, Chichester 1979).

T. P. Hackett, MD, Professor of Psychiatry, Massachusetts General Hospital, Boston, MA 02114 (USA)

Adv. Cardiol., vol. 31, pp. 218–222 (Karger, Basel 1982)

Assessing Psychological Problems from a Cardiologist's Point of View

Joseph E. Acker, Jr., Paula R. MacMorran, James W. Friedlob, Charles C. Wade

Cardiac Rehabilitation Outpatient Programs, Saint Mary's Medical Center and Fort Sanders Presbyterian Hospital, Knoxville, Tenn., USA

In most cardiac rehabilitation programs the cardiologist acts as team leader and coordinates activities including psychological evaluation and management of psychological problems.

The cardiologist is oriented to deal with pathophysiological as well as the normal and pathopsychological sequellae of myocardial infarction (MI) and coronary artery bypass graft (CABG). He acts as coordinator of team activities and as liaison with the primary physician during the rehabilitation program. He may, after consultation with team members and the primary physician, arrange for additional psychological counseling or psychiatric evaluation and treatment.

During routine history and physical and exercise testing the cardiologist may note only the usual anxiety and depression commonly present after MI or CABG. Not infrequently the excessive heart rate or blood pressure response to treadmill testing may suggest anxiety and excessive catecholamine release. Often the patient and spouse (we encourage the spouse to observe the treadmill test) are greatly reassured by favorable response to the treadmill test (TM). Those with excessive heart rate response are observed more closely during early exercise sessions. Occasionally beta-blockers are used to permit higher levels of exercise with more appropriate heart rate (HR) response.

An example of this was B. P., a 64-year-old podiatrist with a recent inferior MI. On initial TM test his HR was 130 at 4 METs, blood pressure (BP) was 180/100, double product 23,400, target heart rate (THR) was set at 115. HR on three successive exercise sessions during warm-up was 116, 112, and 112, and would rise to 130–140 at very low levels of work. Following propranolol 10 mg q.i.d., he was able to exercise at better level for training without exceeding his THR.

Team members and disciplines represented vary with available resources. In one program the clinical specialist skilled in individual, group and family therapy, by structured interview evaluates the psychological and social status of each new patient, and, if possible, the spouse. Group lecture-discussions aimed at life-style changes are the basic approach for our stress management core. Often, however, additional individual counseling with the patient and/or spouse is necessary. Anxiety and depression sufficient to interfere with rehabilitation, difficulty in stopping smoking and sexual problems are frequently helped by additional counseling. Occasionally, drugs are prescribed by the cardiologist after consultation with the primary physician. Rarely, referral to a psychiatrist is necessary. In those rare instances psychiatric problems usually antedate this illness by several years, though masked by a busy life-style.

A.S.C., a 63-year-old who had surgery on the prostate, cervical vertebra, knee, and CABG since 1976 was noted on initial evaluation to be extremely anxious, moderately depressed, a very obsessive, compulsive personality with many somatic complaints. After consultation with the primary physician who prescribed iorazepan (Ativan), symptoms improved dramatically.

One early intervention with perphenazine amitriptyline (Triavil) resulted in an idiosyncratic response of heightened agitation and insomnia. The clinical specialist, atuned to the dynamics of his obsessive compulsive personality attempted to redirect his obsessiveness toward his rehabilitation efforts with much success. He became rather compulsive about practicing with his relaxation tape.

In our other program team members are a medical social worker (MSW) and a clinical psychologist. Initial interview by the MSW brings out social and economic problems. The clinical psychologist uses a test in lieu of an interview. Initially, this was a 16 PF test (personality factors), later a modified Minnesota Multiphasic Personality Inventory (MMPI) called PSI and Activity Preference Questionnaire. Both were discarded as unsatisfactory. During the past year the Jenkins Activity Questionnaire has been more helpful. However, we have found type A and B personality variables to be readily identifiable through a thorough history taking and observation of reactions and interactions within the treatment program. Though this helps classify patients as Friedman type A or B, we are more interested in determining aspects of behavior which the psychologist and patient may attempt to modify. These may be identified in group discussions or individual counseling.

Nurse-Exercise

The nurses who help supervise exercise and coordinate the entire program have previously worked in the Coronary Care Unit (CCU) and in-patient Cardiac Rehabilitation Unit (CRU) programs. They have been trained to look for and manage normal and abnormal psychological problems. Observations may be forwarded to the cardiologist and/or psychologist in written reports. More frequently informal consultation results in appropriate action. Commonly, the nurse observes unusual HR or BP response, marked anxiety of the patient and/or spouse, depression, return-to-work anxieties, evidence of alcohol abuse, or continued smoking, and consults with the team to determine the appropriate intervention.

Group Education and Behavior Modification Sessions

A 30-min group education-behavior modification session precedes each exercise program during the regular 8-week, 24-session Cardiac Rehabilitation Outpatient Program (CROP). One-third of these cover such topics as: (1) a behavioral approach to stopping smoking; (2) sexual rehabilitation; (3) verbal rehearsal and cognitive restructuring; (4) relaxation skills (Benson relaxation response and a progressive muscle relaxation). Much constructive (and occasionally destructive) criticism during group discussion may reveal problems not previously discovered by the cardiologist, nurse, psychologist, or social worker. Peer group pressures or support may frequently solve inappropriate behavior problems. Spouses are encouraged to attend and participate in these group sessions.

Spouses, Other Family Members or Friends

During the exercise sessions spouses usually group together to observe exercises. They frequently leave for a cup of coffee. During this time each spouse is interviewed at least once by the psychiatric nurse or MSW. Conflicts, unusual emotional problems, sexual difficulties, and other problems may be discovered and coped with.

Discussion of mutual fears or problems by the spouses may also continue during the exercise program. Spouses are frequently overly stressed, anxious, depressed, frightened, angry and feel neglected. Our clinical specialist offers an unstructured support group for spouses to address their important needs. The group is open ended and benefits from its 7th and 8th week spouse members who have a lot to offer the new group members. The focus of the spouse group tends to be on their fears and concerns regarding their spouses' cardiac problems, rehabilitation and noncompliance. Frequently, they focus on their anger and accompanying guilt for the burden of the multiple roles they are filling with no support. We are delighted when on rare occasion they are able to focus on areas of interest to them such as hobbies and children, showing a return of interest in themselves and the world around them.

V. G., a 59-year-old with inferior MI, triple vessel disease, not thought to be a surgical candidate, had a rate-related left bundle branch block (LBBB) at HR 115–120 on initial TM test in the absence of pain.

During a spouse group discussion Mrs. G. expressed growing concern over the conflicts between her and her husband. She related that she was becoming hard to live with due to her fear that her husband was doing too much. He would frequently come in the house quite short of breath and remain fatigued throughout the evening. Mrs. G. wanted the staff to intervene but didn't want her husband to know she had expressed concern for fear of worsening the conflict between them.

A routine follow-up session provided the opportunity for the clinical specialist to explore with Mr. G. many aspects of his rehabilitation. During this session she discovered that Mr. G. had assumed that elevated heart rates were only a problem if they were related to physical exertion. Therefore, if he was working on a tedious or emotionally stressful task he would continue for long periods of time, well over his target heart rate. She corrected this misunderstanding and referred him back to the exercise physiologist.

Reinstruction of a very cooperative patient resolved the conflict with the patient staying within his THR. This was especially important since he continued with rate-related BBB in absence of pain on final TM and arm ergometry (AC) tests at HR 110on TM – 120 on AC.

Originally, the regular monthly meetings of CROP group members was planned for administrative problem solving. However, most of each session is spent discussing psychological problems of the patients. Previously unobserved facts brought out by a team member may make management decisions easier. The cardiologist then either carries out decisions or delegates them to the appropriate team member for implementation.

Ambulatory Exercise Monitoring

Each patient has a 24-hour Holter monitor near the end of CROP or after he returns to work. HR response during work, home exercise, and normal daily activities, including sex, are usually well within normal limits.

Occasionally, dysrhythmias are noted. Stress HR responses occasionally occur and can be used to alert the individual to modify his response to the stimulus.

M. C., a 53-year-old male had a quadruple coronary bypass graft in 1977. During Holter monitoring his average high heart rate varied from 85 to 97 but during an argument with his son frequent premature contractions and a heart rate of 136 were noted.

C. W., a successful 57-year-old contractor had a HR of 150 while running in the rain and of 135 while meeting with lawyers and his business partners.

Final Conference

The final conference with patient and spouse coordinates all previous physiological, psychological, and psychosocial parameters. Prescriptions for continuing exercise, stress management, risk factor modification, and work arrangements are discussed. A formal report is mailed to the primary physician for his use.

If the patient continues in an open-ended maintenance program, team members continue to work with each patient indefinitely.

J. E. Acker, Jr., MD, Knoxville Cardiovascular Group P. C., Suite 222, U. T. Physicians Bldg., 1928 Alcoa Hwy, Knoxville, TN 37920 (USA)

Adv. Cardiol., vol. 31, pp. 223–225 (Karger, Basel 1982)

Intensive Care Unit Members in Front of the Patients Reaction Related to an Acute Myocardial Infarction

C. Degré-Coustry, M. Grévisse

Université Libre de Bruxelles, Clinique Cardiologique de l'Hôpital St Pierre, Bruxelles, Belgique

It is commonly accepted that the attitude of patients during their hospitalization is strongly predictive of their return to normal life. Therefore, it is of critical importance that the entire staff in the coronary care unit (CCU) should be aware of the psychological problems of the patients and prepared to handle them in a constructive way. The influence of the nursing staff, which bears consequences on the acceptance of the illness, starts as soon as the patients is taken care of, either at home or at the hospital emergency ward. The psychological problems that patients must face remain identical throughout the illness.

Patient-Specific Problems

All patients with a myocardial infarction admitted to a CCU display anxiety and depressive reactions [2, 5, 6]. Fear of death, pain and the surrounding monitoring equipment are the first sensations of patients who are frequently hospitalized for the first time, in context of pain and emergency. These reactions should be taken into account by the nursing staff and the patient's attitude in facing his illness is judged in terms of possible consequences in the acceptance of the ailment. The psychological evaluation of the patient is essential to allow an adjustment of the nursing staff's attitude.

We studied 304 male patients in working age, hospitalized in a University Hospital CCU of Brussels for myocardial infarction between

1976 and 1979 [4]. After an interview with the patients, they were divided into groups A and B according to the classification of Rosenman and Friedman. They were further divided according to their reaction to the illness as follows:

(1) *Impulsive reaction* (= I): The patient rejects the idea of being ill and minimizes his symptoms. He is aggressive, hyperactive even in the CCU and does not accept restrictions imponed by the nursing staff. His motivation for work remains excellent.

(2) *Adapted reactions* (= A): The patient evaluates the future in a constructive way and is in control of his emotional reactions. He takes CCU restrictions into account. Motivation for work is good.

(3) *Regressive reaction* (= R): The patient is 'overrun' by his emotional reactions, regresses and only reacts by passivity and by dramatizing.

Our criterion of successful rehabilitation was the resumption of professional activities 1 year after myocardial infarction. It is noteworthy that the better the reaction during acute illness in the CCU is, the sooner work is resumed. Contrarily, work resumption becomes more and more difficult if the patient regresses during his hospital stay. Similarly, work resumption is related to the behavioral caracteristics preceding the illness. The closer the patient is to Rosenman and Friedman's type A behavioral pattern, the quicker he resumes work, being disabled by inactivity.

Problems Relating to the Confrontation 'Patient-Environment'

Role of the Family. From the start of hospitalization, the attitude of the family must be investigated. At all levels, the nursing staff should have contacts with the family to assist them in facing a new and unexpected situation. The psychologist and the social worker will help the doctor to adapt the family's behavior towards the patient.

Sexual Problems [1, 7]. From the start of hospitalization, the nursing staff must be prepared to discuss this subject with the patient to avoid the emergence of problems later on.

Modification of Life Habits. The entire nursing staff should help the patient to accept the changes in life habits which have become necessary due to the illness. Knowledge of the patient's reactions is of great importance in this setting.

Conclusion

The entire nursing staff (doctor, nurses, psychologist, social worker, etc.) should be duly informed of the psychology of the patients in order to react constructively during hospitalization, thus allowing a more or less normal resumption of normal life. The staff members should meet and adjust their attitude towards the patient and his family with regard to every individual problem that might arise.

References

1 Bloch, A.; Maeder, J. P.; Haissly, J. C.: Sexual problems after myocardial infarction. Am. Heart J. *90:* 556–537 (1975).

2 Cassem, M. H.; Hackett, T. P.: Psychological rehabilitation of myocardial infarction patient in the acute phase. Heart, Lung *2:* 382–388 (1973).

3 Degré-Coustry, C.: Psychological problems in rehabilitation programs; in Psychological approach to the rehabilitation of coronary patients, pp. 32–34 (Springer, Berlin 1976).

4 Degré-Coustry, C., et al.: Psychological problems in rehabilitation after myocardial infarction: non-institutional approach; in Bund, Adv. Cardiol., vol. 29 (Karger, Basel, in press 1982).

5 Dellipiani, A. W.; Cay, E. L., et al.: Anxiety after a heart attack. Br. Heart J. *38:* 752–757 (1976).

6 Hackett, T. P.; Cassem, N. H.: Psychologic aspects of rehabilitation after myocardial infarction; in Rehabilitation of the coronary Patient, pp. 243–253 (Wiley, New York 1978).

7 Hellerstein, H. K.; Friedman, E. H.: Sexual activity and the post-coronary patient, Archs. intern. Med. *125:* 987–999 (1970).

C. Degré-Coustry, MD, Université Libre de Bruxelles, Clinique Cardiologique de l'Hôpital St Pierre de Bruxelles, B-1000 Bruxelles (Belgium)

Adv. Cardiol., vol. 31, pp. 226–231 (Karger, Basel 1982)

Rehabilitation of Patients after Acute Myocardial Infarction

An Interdisciplinary Family-Oriented Program

Z. Schlesinger, U. Segev

Heart Institute, Assaf Harofe Hospital, Zerifin, Israel;
Tel Aviv University, Tel Aviv, Israel

Introduction

The goal of cardiac rehabilitation is to ensure the recovering post-myocardial infarction (post-MI) patient optimal functioning at work and in the framework of his family and social life. In order to cope with the variant dimensions of cardiac rehabilitation, an ongoing interdisciplinary, family-oriented program was introduced 9 years ago at the Assaf Harofe Hospital, a 700-bed government community hospital in Israel. It is suggested that such a program, which provides physical training, medical follow-up, accurate information, as well as psychological understanding and support, will contribute to the improvement of patients' and their families' way of life. A long-term interdisciplinary, family-oriented cardiac rehabilitation program will be described in this report, along with a short-term one for those unable to take part in the main program.

Structure of the Rehabilitation Program

Team. The interdisciplinary team includes:

(1) A cardiologist as chairman of the team. He is in charge of the medical care and follow-up examinations of the patients. The cardiologist also participates in discussion group meetings with patients and wives, providing them with information about their disease and recommendations concerning various aspects of their lives.

(2) A clinical psychologist who helps patients and their wives to understand and accept the emotional and environmental difficulties and to

Table I. Description of group discussion meetings during first year of rehabilitation program (part I)

Subject	Description	Meetings n	Directed by	Participants
Information and discussion	description of the disease	1	cardiologist	male patients and wives
	risk factors for the development of coronary disease	2	cardiologist and psychologist	
	typical stress conditions for coronary disease	2	cardiologist and psychologist	male patients and wives
	daily behavior guidance	2	cardiologist and psychologist	male patients and wives
	diet and cooking	1	dietician	male patients and wives

Table II. Description of group discussion meetings during first year of rehabilitation program (part II)

Subject	Description	Meetings n	Directed by	Participants
Structured group dynamic meetings for male patients	history of disease and hospitalization (abreaction)	1	psychologist	male patients
	changes in self-image	2	psychologist	male patients
	work relationship and career	2	psychologist	male patients
	family relationships	1	psychologist	male patients
	marital relationships	2	psychologist	male patients
	social and leisure time activities	1	psychologist	male patients

develop techniques in order to cope with them. This work is carried out in group discussion forums.

(3) A licensed physiotherapist who helps the patients, in a group setting, to master relaxation techniques and, through an intensive exercise program, to improve their physical fitness.

(4) A nurse coordinator who is in charge of the regular functioning of the program. Also, through her personal contact with the patients, she is often the first to notice any physical or psychological changes and brings them to the attention of the rehabilitation team.

Table III. Description of group discussion meetings during first year of rehabilitation program (part III)

Subject	Description	Meetings n	Directed by	Participants
Structured group dynamic meetings for patients' wives	acceptance of the disease (abreaction)	1	psychologist	patients' wives
	how to help the spouse	2	cardiologist	patients' wives
	wives' fears und conflicts and how to deal with them	2	psychologist	patients' wives
Summary	planning personal and family way of life for future	2	cardiologist and psychologist	patients and wives
	towards summer vacation	1	cardiologist and psychologist	patients and wives

(5) A dietician who helps patients to plan their diet habits. The whole team has regular staff meetings which enable coordination and establish an atmosphere of an interdisciplinary team project.

Patients. The program was started in April 1972 with 25 male patients. Each year a new group with about the same number of patients joined the program. By January 1981, ten groups totaling 260 patients, aged 35–65, had taken part in the program. The criteria for selecting post-MI patients for this program were as follows:

All patients had experienced an acute MI proven by electrocardiographic evidence and repeated blood enzyme examination. None of these patients had congestive heart failure, marked angina pectoris or severe rhythm disturbances. In order to take part in the program all patients had to be interviewed to determine their motivations and intellectual abilities.

Rehabilitation Schedule. The rehabilitation program is divided into two main periods:

(a) The first year: The first 3 months of the rehabilitation program comprise three group meetings per week, each lasting 1 h. The majority of the exercises during this period are performed in the supine position and include mainly relaxation and respiratory exercises. The initial period is followed by the regular prolonged rehabilitation program which includes two group meetings of 1 h each per week. These meetings are mainly aimed at improving physical fitness. During the entire period, patients and their

Table IV. Follow-up meetings for patients participating in the rehabilitation program for more than 1 year

Subject	Description	Meetings n	Directed by	Participants
Information and discussion	risk factors	1	cardiologist and psychologist	male patients and wives
	open discussion based on questions	2	cardiologist and psychologist	male patients and wives
	discussion focused on readjustment to work	1	cardiologist and psychologist	male patients and wives
	discussion focused on family difficulties	2	cardiologist and psychologist	male patients and wives
	discussion focused on day-to-day difficulties	1	cardiologist and psychologist	male patients and wives

wives meet with members of the rehabilitation team for group discussions. The group meets once every 2 weeks for 60 min (table I–III).

(b) The second and successive years: Advanced physical exercises, such as calisthenics, jogging, ball games, etc., are administered for 1 h twice a week in order to improve patients' cardiovascular fitness. Six group discussion meetings for patients and their wive are scheduled for the year (table IV). The second-year program is repeated during the following year. The patients are allowed to stay with program as long as they wish.

After 9 years of experience, it can be concluded that a slow stream of dropping out starts after the first year. About 50% of the patients continue to the third year and only a few remain for the fourth and following years. Each year three groups are operated simultaneously: one group of 25 first-year patients and two groups of about 30 patients each who decided to remain in the program. During the entire program, individual medical, psychological and psychiatric treatment is available when required.

Group Discussions with Patients

Group discussion meetings are designed to help patients cope with personal and environmental difficulties resulting from the need to adjust to their new status as heart patients. In order to do so we deal with two main dimensions of the patients' lives:

Information. After leaving the hospital, heart patients are exposed to myths and popular misconceptions about their prospective life expectancy, desirable and undesirable behavior and the demands they are justified in making on their families, friends and colleagues at work. The unreliability and inconsistency of this information creates confusion, conflicts, and thereby, feelings of insecurity. Restrictive advice on how to deal with this information may create anxiety which may lead to uncooperative behavior. Regular and informal group meetings with a cardiologist and psychologist help to reduce anxiety and create a goal-oriented atmosphere.

Personal and Family Dynamics. In order to provide patients with the opportunity to raise and confront emotional and environmental difficulties, psychodynamic group meetings are arranged. Most patients begin this part of the program with abreactive responses (the process of releasing a repressed emotion by reliving in imagination the original experience) to the existential trauma they had experienced with the MI and hospitalization in the intensive coronary care unit. Following the abreactive stage, each group related to almost the same subjects which represented the major areas of readjustment difficulties. Major subjects raised within the group discussion are:

– Changes of the division of roles in the family (the wife assumes many of the roles which had been the husband's responsibility).

– Many patients faced a dependence-independence conflict in their relationship with their wives. They searched for a way to deal with the helpful and sometimes overprotective wife while still remaining independent.

– The future of the family unit became unclear. Young patients especially (but not exclusively) felt they had disappointed familial expectations for a safe and better future.

– Sex became an area of stress due to fear of death. Masculinity, under these circumstances, became ambiguous and questioned.

– Relationships with young children were conflictual. For many young patients, feelings of guilt, inadequacy and disappointment, and at the same time desire for respect, resulted in tension in the paternal-filial relationship.

Short-Term Rehabilitation Program

The above-described rehabilitation program has its limitations, to some of which we found a solution by creating a model short-term rehabilitation program. The major limitations of the long-term program

Table V. Abbreviated rehabilitation program schedule for ten meetings

Subject	Description	Meetings n	Directed by	Participants
Information and discussion	description of the disease	1	cardiologist	male patients and wives
	risk factors	2	cardiologist and psychologist	male patients and wives
	discussion on diet and cooking	1	dietician	male patients and wives
	guidance for daily behavior	1	cardiologist and psychologist	male patients and wives
	family and sexual life	2	psychologist	male patients and wives
	recommended occupational activities	1	cardiologist and psychologist	male patients and wives
	typical stress conditions	1	cardiologist and psychologist	male patients and wives
	social and leisure time activities	1	cardiologist and psychologist	male patients and wives

are: (a) It deals only with male patients. An effort must be made to help women after an acute MI and their families. (b) Only a select group of patients can take advantage of the program: They must be medically fit to take part in the physical exercises. In addition they must have motivation and the technical means to reach the out-of-town hospital twice a week in all conditions of weather. These conditions are correlated with a relatively high socioeconomic status.

The short-term rehabilitation program (table V) is based on relaxation techniques and information sessions. It demands only ten meetings of 90 min each to which patients and their wives are encouraged to come. The program begins as soon as possible after the patient's discharge from the hospital, and no more than 3 months afterwards. This arrangement does not interfere with the patient's occupational obligations. It is also short enough to prevent dropping out as a result of environmental, psychological or economic pressures.

Z. Schlesinger, MD, Heart Institute, Assaf Harofe Hospital, 70300 Zerifin (Israel)

Adv. Cardiol., vol. 31, pp. 232–236 (Karger, Basel 1982)

Measuring the Outcome of Rehabilitation

Alistair E. Philip

Department of Clinical Psychology, Royal Edinburgh Hospital, Edinburgh, UK

Studies carried out in a number of centres [1, 3, 5, 7, 11] have established the importance of psychological and social factors in recovery and subsequent rehabilitation after a myocardial infarction. These studies have typically demonstrated significant relationships between psychosocial variables and outcome, either by correlations or by group differences, but have differed greatly in the range and kind of psychosocial and outcome measures reported. A report by *Philip* et al. [8] has demonstrated the value of applying multivariate statistical techniques to psychosocial data; unimportant variables can be discarded and the efficacy of measures which do not depend on research staff or specialised techniques can be ascertained. Similar methods of analysis can be applied to the problem of outcome.

It is difficult to select any one measure of outcome of recovery after myocardial infarction. Death is clearly an unsatisfactory outcome but so also is being alive but severely restricted and handicapped by the residual effects of the acute episode. Being alive is a necessary condition for a satisfactory outcome, but just being alive is not a sufficient condition for good outcome. In many countries return to work, with its attendant economic, social and physical implications, has been viewed as a useful, practical measure of outcome. Current trends in world-wide unemployment have severely restricted the utility of return to work as an index of outcome. The study of *Philip* et al. [8] used a number of physical, psychological and social variables as outcome measures of equal validity, acknowledging that the relative validities of these measures required detailed study. This paper attempts such a study, using the statistical method of multivariate analysis known as factor analysis [6].

The purpose of factor analysis is to explain the observed relationships among a relatively large number of variables in terms of a smaller set of relationships. Most measures of outcome correlate with one another to a greater or lesser degree and the number of correlations increases rapidly with the addition of a few more variables, in fact n variables yield ½n (n-1) non-redundant correlations. Thus, 5 variables produce 10 correlations, 10 variables produce 45 correlations whilst 15 variables will generate 105 correlations. Factor analysis and related methods reduce the complexity of such large sets of correlations and make it easier for the human mind to grasp the nature of the underlying relationships and to integrate this new information with existing knowledge and theory. The practising clinician need not be concerned about the algebraic and computing aspects of factor analysis. Conceptually, a factor analysis starts by collecting scores on tests or performance ratings of individuals, transforming such scores into a table of correlations between the tests or ratings and then transforming these correlations into a table of 'factor loadings' or correlations between the tests and a small number of mathematically abstracted factors.

Method

The patients studied have not been reported upon previously. Of 275 consecutive male admissions to the Coronary Care Unit of the Royal Infirmary of Edinburgh, 197 were sufferers of a first myocardial infarction. 1 year later 18 patients were known to be dead and of the 179 survivors 160 (89%) came to a follow-up clinic where they were reviewed independently by a physician and a psychiatrist.

The physician graded each patient's symptoms of angina and breathlessness according to the WHO criteria [9], recorded the occurrence of ischaemic attacks, the use of drugs (GTN, beta blockers, digoxin, tranquillisers) and ascertained the patient's current level of exercise compared with the level before infarction. Physical examination established the presence or absence of heart murmurs, evidence of cardiac failure, blood pressure and weight. An ECG recording and a chest X-ray were carried out to ascertain any left ventricular failure and to establish the cardio-thoracic ratio.

The psychiatrist assessed the patient's current emotional state using *Goldberg's* [2] structured interview, established whether the patient was working and if work was at the same level of activity as before. She also recorded the patient's own assessment of his degree of physical disability and monitored the completion of two psychological tests, the General Health Questionnaire [2] and Form D of the Eight Parallel Form Anxiety Questionnaire [10].

The scores and ratings on these 21 variables were correlated and then factor analysed using a standard computer program [4].

Table I. Varimax rotated factors: loadings on outcome measures

Outcome variables	Factors I	II	III	IV	V	VI	VII	VIII
Work status	144	134	588	–080	230	051	–083	010
Activity at work	081	164	567	–028	033	036	–014	083
Rating of emotional upset	458	091	326	040	235	065	–152	199
Physical disability	358	315	211	186	359	269	054	128
General Health Questionnaire	922	243	153	–056	–027	077	013	–115
Cattell anxiety	447	–076	049	081	066	–057	161	207
Weight	060	031	–114	096	–063	–667	–202	–025
Angina	137	559	307	119	009	087	053	299
Ischaemia	126	420	–025	–056	147	–056	048	–080
Breathlessness	094	183	156	–033	723	018	045	033
GTN	–040	501	196	063	062	–074	–013	237
Beta blockers	257	245	110	–185	129	–020	444	–114
Digoxin	–017	072	270	328	–129	271	019	–065
Tranquillisers	324	084	–061	–089	084	116	099	262
Exercise	035	551	111	077	037	150	021	–173
Heart murmurs	–104	106	077	468	–021	–008	248	048
Cardiac failure	106	034	–027	027	001	274	–116	073
X-ray for LVF	–013	004	–005	415	–012	–061	–057	–057
ECG for LVF	052	–025	–257	200	–038	062	526	121
Cardio-thoracic ratio	089	–004	–224	474	050	044	006	023
Diastolic BP	073	–011	051	–023	011	049	004	393

For clarity the decimal point preceding each value has been omitted.

Results

The results of the factor analysis are shown in table I. A total of eight factors are required to represent the complex relationships between the 21 variables. Four of the factors are of minor importance; factors V, VI and VIII each contain only one factor loading which meets the usual criteria for significance so that these factors can be equated with the original variables of breathlessness, weight and blood pressure, respectively. Factor VII has moderately high loadings or correlations with two outcome measures, ECG for left ventricular failure and use of beta blockers.

The remaining factors (I–IV) each have loadings or correlations with two or more outcome variables which satisfy very stringent criteria for significance. For factor I these key variables are the General Health

Questionnaire, psychiatrist's rating of emotional upset and Cattell Anxiety. This factor is readily interpretable as tapping the psychological aspects of outcome. Factor II contains four key variables, angina, amount of exercise, use of GTN and ischaemia and can be identified as a factor of physical well being at follow up. Factor III reflects performance at work, the key outcome variables being work status and activity at work. The three key variables associated with factor IV, cardio-thoracic ratio, heart murmurs and X-ray evidence of left ventricular failure, identify this factor as being concerned with demonstrable cardiac pathology.

Discussion

These results demonstrate that outcome for survivors of a myocardial infarction has four main aspects. In general, these facts reflect what has been known, the physical, psychological and social aspects of outcome must be examined separately. What has not been known is how best to assess these aspects, using as few measures as possible. Nor has it been previously demonstrated that physical well being in general should be assessed separately from evidence of cardiac pathology.

The methods used to measure outcome must be robust enough to be used in any cardiology department by staff who have no special training in psychological measurement and who may have no access to complicated, expensive physiological instruments. The factors reported in this paper can be represented by such robust measures while, equally, more elaborate investigations, both physical and psychological, can be incorporated within the same conceptual framework.

For routine clinical monitoring of the patient's emotional state the General Health Questionnaire is both a robust measure and a good index of factor I. Clearly, any cardiology department with a psychologist on its staff could use other measures and would be able to examine the contribution of other personality traits to outcome. However, even these departments could use the General Health Questionnaire so as to relate their findings to those of other centres.

The presence of angina, moderated by the use of drugs such as GTN, is a robust measure of general physical well being. As with factor I, such robust measures can be reported routinely without detriment to the development of more precise measures such as exercise tolerance tests and the like. New techniques of cardiac investigation such as catheterisation, angiography and echo-cardiography can add precision to the appraisal of cardiac pathology but simple methods, such as X-ray and the use of a stethescope, will continue to be valid for most purposes.

The social aspects of outcome are the most difficult to measure in a way which can transcend differences between centres. It was stated earlier that work can no longer be viewed as a dependable index of social rehabilitation but it may have to remain in use for some time to come. Economic, cultural and political differences all impinge on social outcome to an extent which is much greater than their effect on the other areas identified.

References

1 Cay, E. L.; Vetter, N. J.; Philip, A. E.; Dugard, P.: Return to work after a heart attack. J. psychosom. Res. *16:* 231–243 (1973).

2 Goldberg, D. P.: The detection of psychiatric illness by questionnaire (Oxford University Press, London 1972).

3 Nagle, R.; Gangola, R.; Picton-Robinson, I.: Factors influencing return to work after myocardial infarction. Lancet *ii:* 454–456 (1971).

4 Nie, N. H.; Hull, C. H.; Jenkins, J. G.; Stenbrenner, K.; Bent, D. H.: Statistical package for the social sciences; 2nd ed. (McGraw-Hill, New York 1975).

5 Pancheri, P.; Bella Terra, M.; Matteoli, S.; Cristofari, M.; Polizzi, C.; Puletti, M.: Infarct as a stress agent. Life history and personality characteristics in improved versus not improved patients after severe heart attack. J. hum. Stress *4:* 16–22, 41–42 (1978).

6 Philip, A. E.; McCulloch, J. W.; Smith, N. J.: Social work research and the analysis of social data, pp. 165–188 (Pergamon, Oxford 1975).

7 Philip, A. E.; Cay, E. L.; Vetter, N. J.; Stuckey, N. A.: Personal traits and the physical, psychiatric and social state of patients one year after a myocardial infarction. Int. J. Rehab. Res. *2:* 479–487 (1979).

8 Philip, A. E.; Cay, E. L.; Stuckey, N. A.; Vetter, N. J.: Multiple predictors and multiple outcome after myocardial infarction. J. psychosom. Res. *25:* 137–141 (1981).

9 Rose, G. A.; Blackburn, H.: Cardiovascular population studies. Methods (WHO, Geneva 1966).

10 Scheier, I. H.; Cattell, R. B.: Handbook for the IPAT 8-parallel form anxiety battery (IPAT, Champaign 1960).

11 Wynn, A.: Unwarranted emotional distress in men with ischaemic heart disease. Med. J. Aust. *ii:* 847–851 (1967).

Dr. A. E. Philip, Department of Clinical Psychology, Royal Edinburgh Hospital, Morningside Terrace, Edinburgh, EH10 5HF (UK)

Adv. Cardiol., vol. 31, pp. 237–241 (Karger, Basel 1982)

Psychological Aspects of Cardiac Rehabilitation

Unsolved Problems

Elizabeth L. Cay

Rehabilitation Medicine Unit, Astley Ainslie Hospital, and the Rehabilitation Studies Unit, University of Edinburgh, Edinburgh, UK

Although many studies have shown that various kinds of rehabilitation programmes for patients after myocardial infarction have undoubted physical and psychological benefits, many physicians remain sceptical of their value. They point out that three recent multicentre studies have failed to demonstrate that rehabilitation, mainly based on exercise, results in a decrease in mortality or further infarction.

The American National Exercise and Heart Disease Project reported significant physiological and psychological improvement in 651 post-infarct patients during a pre-randomised low level programme but the organisers now doubt that a definitive answer will be forthcoming because of small sample size and inadequate length of follow-up. *Shephard* [this volume] has reported some of the results of the Ontario Multicentre Exercise Heart Trial involving 751 post-infarct patients. 51 had another infarct in the course of the study, almost half of them related to some form of exercise. The majority of episodes occurred in individuals who did not attend the programme regularly or who had evidence of severe myocardial damage on exercise testing. For the first time, *Shephard* formally raised the question that the aim of reducing mortality or preventing another infarction may be asking too much of a rehabilitation programme. More attention should be paid to its influence on the quality of life during the patient's remaining years. The results of the WHO European Multicentre Study of the effect of comprehensive rehabilitation, due to be published shortly, would seem to support this view. There was no difference overall in death or recurrence of infarction between rehabilitation and control groups. Despite uncontrolled and subjective methods of assessing anxiety, depression and social problems, the results do suggest that the rehabilitation group adjusted more

Table I. Return to work after a myocardial infarction related to emotional disturbance

Severity of upset	Patients working %	Working as hard as before %
None	77	74
Mild	69	36
Severe	57	20

quickly and had fewer social problems a year after their infarct than the control group with the difference disappearing by the end of 3 years.

It appears that those of us working in the field of rehabilitation, convinced at a clinical level of its value, will have to define clearly what is meant by a 'good' outcome if we are to influence our colleagues. It is relatively easy to assess psychological and social problems and their effect on outcome, particularly if one aspect, namely return to work, is chosen as the outcome measure (table I). Working efficiency following an infarct drops with increasing severity of emotional disturbance. Of some 200 male patients, 1 in 4 were still quite severely distressed 4 months after their infarct. These patients did badly; just over half went back to work but only 20% were working as hard as before. It is much more difficult if outcome embraces a variety of physical, psychological and social factors, the quality of a patient's life after his illness. Yet, this is obviously the only realistic way to judge success or failure of rehabilitation and will become increasingly important in the future if, as seems possible, work will fill our lives to a lesser extent than at present.

Measurement of a diverse variety of outcomes is easy in large centres with access to specially trained staff who have time to devote to research. The challenge for the future is to develop methods of handling these 'soft' data which are suitable for use on a service basis in any busy cardiological department or district general hospital.

Approximately three quarters of patients do well following an infarct provided they are given active encouragement from the beginning of illness (table II). The others do badly, not that they have had more severe heart attacks, but because they are anxious and depressed, are unable to cope and have related social problems. The 'worst' patients in this respect can be identified early. It is tempting to select this proportion for special rehabilitation efforts. But there is evidence that they may not be the ones who benefit most from a rehabilitation programme; 58% of a group of 197 male

Table II. Return to work related to initial reaction to an infarction (% of patients)

Emotional upset 5–8 days after myocardial infarction	Return to full activity by 4 months	Return to full activity within 1 year
Absent	52	88
Present	36	31

Table III. Outcome 1 year after a first myocardial infarction (% of patients)

	Good risk	Bad risk
Work		
Working as hard	58	50
Working less well	32	24
Not working	10	26
Emotional upset		
None	40	16
Mild	43	44
Moderate	17	40

patients following a first infarction were identified as bad risks on account of emotional upset and/or social problems (table III). On the whole the bad risks did less well then the others but quite a number of the good risks had not done as well as expected. It appears that the criteria of those likely to benefit most from a rehabilitation programme are not yet properly defined, an important consideration for all those involved in the cost of delivering health care services. Should we be concentrating our rehabilitation efforts in those with less severe upset and minor social problems?

Adjustment after an infarct is not static. Even in the first week or two there are considerable fluctuations in anxiety (fig. 1). In a group of over 400 consecutive admissions to a coronary care unit in a Scottish hospital, anxiety was high when they were tested on average half an hour after admission. After a transitory rise in anxiety on transfer from the unit, they settled quickly in the ward becoming almost euphoric as discharge home became imminent. Too precipitate a selection in this group would have meant that too many patients would have been identified as likely to do badly while if selection had been delayed too long too few would have been

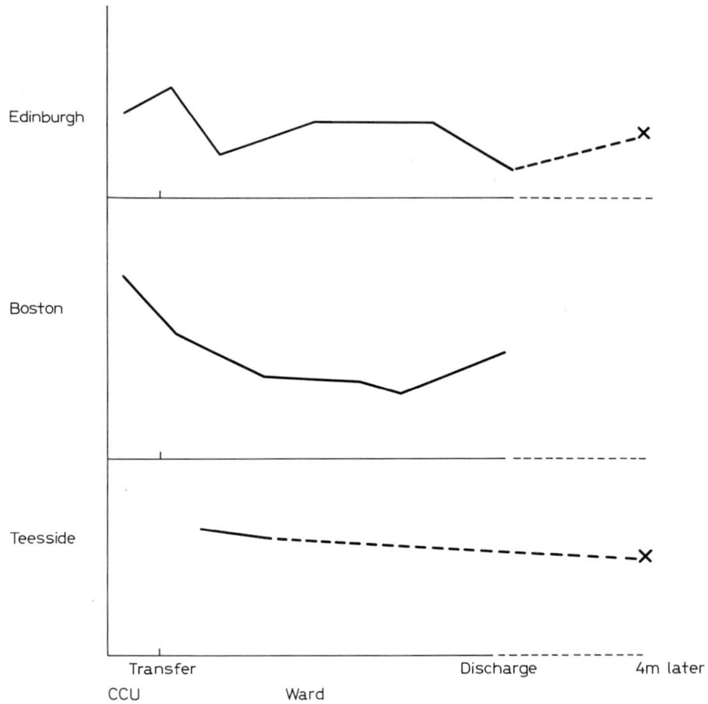

Fig. 1. Anxiety after a myocardial infarction. CCU = Coronary care unit.

picked out. the 'best' timc appeared to be 5–8 days after transfer from the coronary care unit. This is not necessarily applicable to all patients after an infarct; anxiety measured in the same way was much higher in another group from an industrialized area in North England not 100 miles distant. Patients in a Boston hospital in *Hackett's* series had quite a different pattern of anxiety during the acute phase of illness; they tended, possibly more realistically than the Edinburgh patients, to anticipate the problems facing them after they left hospital. There is obviously considerable need to try to find out when patients should be selected for a rehabilitation programme. Is it possible to do this with simple practical methods which could be used in more than one centre?

Many different kinds of rehabilitation programme have been described. They may be in-patient or out-patient, based on a rehabilitation centre, teaching or general hospital or within the community. They vary in length from one session to several sessions per week lasting for weeks, months or years and start at different times after the onset of infarction. Relations may or may not be included and though there is general agreement that rehabilitation should be comprehensive there is considerable individual variation in the type of programme offered. While each has its protagonists and antagonists there is as yet no definite evidence on which type of programme gives the best results. Nor do we know which component of a comprehensive scheme of rehabilitation is of benefit.

Until very recently doctors and therapists have tended to believe that giving advice to patients means that they will understand what they are told and that they will follow instructions. A few studies have begun to demonstrate that this is not always the case. *Jackson* who reported on 24 patients after an infarct, 14 of whom were given a simple written guide to take home with them in addition to routine verbal advice, found that understanding of the disease and resumption of sexual activity was significantly better in those who had received the written guide. There is need of more studies like this to evaluate different types of cardiac rehabilitation, particularly their effect on the adjustment of patient and family to life after an infarct.

On the whole, substantial beneficial changes have been reported following cardiac rehabilitation programmes. Most deal with short-term outcomes, variously defined. Are these changes sustained or is the long-term outcome unaltered? These are but a few examples of some of the unsolved problems in this very complicated area. The prospect of finding answers is daunting but must be undertaken if physicians as a whole are to be convinced that attention to the patient's emotional well-being is an integral part of patient care and not, as many view it, a luxurious extra.

E. L. Cay, MD, Rehabilitation Medicine Unit, Astley Ainslie Hospital,
Grange Loan, Edinburgh EH9 2HL (UK)

Subject Index

Aerobic requirements 187
Ambulation early 147
  accelerated vs. 152
  cardiac mortality during 144
  CCU stay 143
  complications 143
  high risk patient 145
  ward stay 143
Ambulatory exercise monitoring 221
Angina pectoris
  physical training 186, 191
  prognosis 191
  stable 46, 65
  unstable 47, 67
Anginal pain, relief 192
Anticoagulants 116
  long-term study 99
  secondary prevention 98
Anturane Reinfarction Trial 100
  sudden death reduction 100
Aortocoronary bypass surgery 150
  exercise testing 28, 31
  exercise tolerance 73
  functional status improvement 81
  indications 45, 49, 60
  premature mortality 51
  secondary prevention 60
  survival, long-term 57, 81
  symptom status improvement 81
Arrhythmias, ventricular 144, 206
  control 115
  myocardial infarction after 38
  suppression 70
Aspirin Myocardial Infarction Study 100
  reinfarction 100
A-V oxygen difference 188

Bayes theorem 4, 14, 20
Beta-blocking drugs 117, 188, 207
  hypertensive patients 97
  value of therapy 87, 88, 90
Blood pressure control 171
Bypass surgery 117
  enhancement of survival 81
  working status after 75–78

Calcium blockers 86
Cardiac energy expenditure, decrease 194
Cardiac output
  decrease 195
  maximal exercise 189
Catecholamines 182
Chest pain, atypical 9
Congestive heart failure 47
Coronary angiography, infarction
  predictor 24
Coronary artery disease
  diagnosis 5
  double vessel disease 63
  ejection fraction 25
  left main artery 63
  prevalence 5

Coronary artery disease
triple vessel disease 63
Coronary blood flow
increase 192
redistribution 194
Coronary circulation, trained animals 181
Coronary Drug Project 162
Coronary mortality
Belgian study 104
early ambulation during 144
Finnish study 126
WHO study 109
Coronary score 30
Coronary spasm 48
Cycle length 193

Deconditioning, complications 140

Ear densitography, STI monitoring 36
ECG interpretation
myocardial infarction 148
reliability 15
Echocardiography 181
Ectopy, ventricular
exercise-induced 43
prognostic significance 42
Ejection fraction 205
left main artery disease 25
prognostic importance 24
proximal three-vessel disease 25, 26
Ergometry bicycle 158, 159, 182
European Coronary Surgery Study
52–56, 82
Exercise ECG
angiography relation 2
coronary artery disease prevalence 5
diagnostic accuracy 4
Exercise programming 208, 209
Exercise testing
aortocoronary bypass surgery 23, 30
asymptomatic patients 48
clinical implications 1
false-negative results 15, 20
false-positive results 15, 20
limitations 20
post-myocardial infarction 42
predictive accuracy 3, 16
prognostic value 6, 10, 12, 20, 23, 28, 38
results definition 2
screening protocol 13
sensitivity 3, 13, 21
specificity 3, 13
submaximal 159
symptom-limited 159
Exercise therapy 135
value 191
Exercise tolerance after coronary surgery 74
Exercise training, vigorous 199, 205

Finnish study
mortality 124, 125
reinfarction 126
Functional capacity, myocardial infarction, following 160

Heart rate
maximal 131
reserve 131
perceived exertion 132
submaximal 159
Hypertension 177
control 116, 171
treatment 96, 97
Hypotension, orthostatic 139

Infarct size 181
reduction 87
Ischemic heart disease, prevention 95

Left ventricular ejection time (LVET) 36
Left ventricular function 158
improvement 67
Lipid lowering drugs 163
Lipids, exercise 172, 178, 201

Master two-step test, augmented 12
Maximal oxygen uptake 139, 189
Metoprolol study 87
infarct size reduction 93
mortality 93
Myocardial contractility, changes 195
Myocardial infarction
acceleration 153, 154

Myocardial infarction
acute beta blockade 91
anxiety after 240
depression after 215
early ambulation after 138, 142, 147
emotional upset after 239
exercise testing 9
physiologic impairment after 202
psychological and social factors 232
reconditioning after 156, 157
rehabilitation after 226
secondary prevention after 86
work status 234
Myocardial oxygen extraction, increase 194

New York Heart Association, functional classification 108, 202, 203
coronary surgery 61
Newcastle study 164
Non-invasive techniques 1, 181
North Karelia project 122
mortality 123
reinfarction 123

Ontario Exercise and Heart Collaborative Study 104

Patient compliance 134
Patient education 215, 220, 228–231
behaviour modification 220
family role 224
life habits 224
sexual problems 224
PEP/LVET 36
Perceived exertion 132
Perfext 182
Persantin Aspirin Reinfarction Study 100
mortality 100
Physical activity 114
benefits 203
strenuous 199
Physical conditioning, myocardial infarction, following 156
Physical training
adherence 188
animal study 181
blood pressure 173, 178, 181
comparison of methods 131
goals 200
hemodynamic changes 182, 187
high-density lipoprotein 172
intensity 129
low-density lipoprotein 172
myocardial infarction after 107
perceived exertion 129
physiological response 200
prescription 201
Physical work capacity 135, 139, 173, 200
Platelet-active agents, secondary prevention 99
Preejection period (PEP)
coronary angiography 36
sensitivity 37
Prevention of coronary heart disease
primary 112, 162
secondary 113, 120, 134, 163
Propranolol 87, 188, 207, 208
Psychological aspects
denial 213
misconceptions 214
rehabilitation 212, 218, 222, 226, 237
relaxation techniques 216
tranquilizers 216
Psychosocial stress 115
Pulmonary ventilation 140

Quality of life 122

Radionuclide testing methods 23, 182, 184
angiography 24
severe CAD prediction 25
Randomized trials 134, 169
Rate pressure product 135, 187, 194, 200
Rehabilitation
community approach 120
comprehensive 103, 135, 156
early 102, 138, 142, 152, 206
accelerated 153, 154
interdisciplinary program 226
outcome measures 234
procedure, coronary bypass surgery 80
program, short-term 230

Rehabilitation
psychological aspects
212, 218, 222, 226, 237
psychological effect 135
risk factor modification 170
vocational, coronary surgery after
75–77, 83
Return to work 201, 238, 239
Risk factors 135
modification 168, 176, 201
R wave alternation 2, 148

Sexual orgasm, sudden death 215
Smoking habits 165, 170, 173, 177
coronary mortality 165
reinfarction 165
ST segment depression 157, 200
after coronary surgery 74
hypertensive men 9
Stroke volume 135, 188
Sudden cardiac death 96
coronary artery disease 70
exercise testing 9
Symptom-limited testing 8
Systolic time intervals 32
exercise response 35
prognostic value 35, 46

Thallium scintigraphy 20, 24, 158, 182
Thrombo-embolic complications 140
Tranquilizers, use 216
Treadmill testing 157, 158
Tymolol study 87, 93

US National Exercise and Heart Disease
Project 104, 168

Ventricular arrhythmias 144, 206
exercise effect 201
exercise-induced 38
prognostic significance 39

Wall tension, changes 193
WHO Collaborative Study 107, 237
mortality 109
reinfarction 110